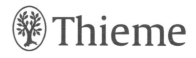

Atlas of Full-Endoscopic Spine Surgery

Christoph P. Hofstetter, MD, PhD, FACS
Associate Professor
Department of Neurological Surgery
University of Washington Medical Center
Seattle, Washington

Sebastian Ruetten, MD
Attending Spine Surgeon
Center for Spine Surgery and Pain Therapy
Center for Orthopaedics and Traumatology
of the St. Elisabeth Group – Catholic Hospital Rhein-Ruhr
St. Anna Hospital Herne/Marien Hospital Herne University Hospital/Marien Hospital Witten
Herne, Germany

Yue Zhou, MD, PhD
Professor
Department of Orthopaedics
Xinqiao Hospital
Army Medical University
Chongqing, China

Michael Y. Wang, MD, FACS
Professor
Departments of Neurosurgery and Rehab Medicine
University of Miami School of Medicine
Miami, Florida

Illustrations in this book were supported with grants from Joimax® and Storz.

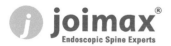

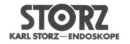

488 illustrations

Thieme
New York • Stuttgart • Delhi • Rio de Janeiro

Library of Congress Cataloging-in-Publication Data is available from the publisher

Thieme Publishers New York
333 Seventh Avenue, New York, NY 10001 USA
+1 800 782 3488, customerservice@thieme.com

Georg Thieme Verlag KG
Rüdigerstrasse 14, 70469 Stuttgart, Germany
+49 [0]711 8931 421, customerservice@thieme.de

Thieme Publishers Delhi
A-12, Second Floor, Sector-2, Noida-201301
Uttar Pradesh, India
+91 120 45 566 00, customerservice@thieme.in

Thieme Publishers Rio de Janeiro
Thieme Publicações Ltda.
Edifício Rodolpho de Paoli, 25º andar
Av. Nilo Peçanha, 50 – Sala 2508
Rio de Janeiro 20020-906 Brasil
+55 21 3172 2297

Cover design: Thieme Publishing Group
Typesetting by Thomson Digital, India

Printed in Germany by Beltz Grafische Betriebe   5 4

ISBN 978-1-68420-023-8

Also available as an e-book:
eISBN 978-1-68420-024-5

Important note: Medicine is an ever-changing science undergoing continual development. Research and clinical experience are continually expanding our knowledge, in particular our knowledge of proper treatment and drug therapy. Insofar as this book mentions any dosage or application, readers may rest assured that the authors, editors, and publishers have made every effort to ensure that such references are in accordance with **the state of knowledge at the time of production of the book.**

Nevertheless, this does not involve, imply, or express any guarantee or responsibility on the part of the publishers in respect to any dosage instructions and forms of applications stated in the book. **Every user is requested to examine carefully** the manufacturers' leaflets accompanying each drug and to check, if necessary in consultation with a physician or specialist, whether the dosage schedules mentioned therein or the contraindications stated by the manufacturers differ from the statements made in the present book. Such examination is particularly important with drugs that are either rarely used or have been newly released on the market. Every dosage schedule or every form of application used is entirely at the user's own risk and responsibility. The authors and publishers request every user to report to the publishers any discrepancies or inaccuracies noticed. If errors in this work are found after publication, errata will be posted at www.thieme.com on the product description page.

Some of the product names, patents, and registered designs referred to in this book are in fact registered trademarks or proprietary names even though specific reference to this fact is not always made in the text. Therefore, the appearance of a name without designation as proprietary is not to be construed as a representation by the publisher that it is in the public domain.

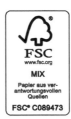

To my family, mentors, fellows, and residents

As to diseases, make a habit of two things—to help, or at least, to do no harm.

Hippocrates

Contents

Contents

Foreword

This edition is special. Professor Hofstetter's *Atlas of Full-Endoscopic Spine Surgery* is a contribution that represents the leading edge of spine surgery. Endoscopic spine surgery is incredibly attractive to both surgeons and patients because of the predictably laudable outcomes and an enviable rapid patient recovery window for a spectrum of pathology. In our surgical armamentarium, this volume's significance is far more than a mere contemporary overview of the burgeoning field of endoscopic spine surgery.

This 26-chapter compendium is written with a remarkable surgical flair. It is thorough, comprehensible, and efficient. It is a step-by-step, concise description written for a broad range of learners, from those fully trained to those still part of the training phase. It is shaped by renowned surgeons who have helped push this evolving endoscopic spine field forward. Most of the chapters are penned by the editor who has an intuitive ability to communicate the most challenging surgical aspects of each operation to even a novice surgeon.

The photographs, drawings, figures, and writing style of this atlas are exceptional in nature, as there is not a single wasted stroke, figure, or chapter. The authors thought of everything from radiation safety to perioperative care. Especially, the surgical techniques chapters, which are simply a cut above many other spine atlas offerings. The atlas offers pearls, practical surgical considerations, and brilliant illustrations of how to deliver an endoscopic surgical solution.

The descriptions are almost mathematical in their emphasis on trajectories, three-dimensional anatomical perspective, and essential psychomotor nuances. The author meticulously describes everything from the position of the surgeon's hands to the anatomical landmarks, as viewed through the endoscope. This is accomplished with the help of beautiful, crystal-clear endoscopic photographs coupled with perfectly choreographed perspectives of the patient/surgeon interface.

Each chapter of this all-encompassing atlas has been crafted intelligently and logically to successfully guide the surgeon through an endoscopic spine procedure. In essence, the atlas is framed in a style that reflects how we, as surgeons, think, analyze, and execute a surgical plan when treating patients with spine conditions. Professor Hofstetter's atlas helps elevate the subject matter to the impeccable technical standards of other classic, academic brain and spine surgery-related subject matter. In addition, the book incorporates the AO nomenclature that will be the basis for the AO worldwide teaching curriculum. Finally, it will likely standardize endoscopic techniques to allow surgeons to compare their results, as this field grows exponentially.

This is a "must have" book for surgeons who are committed to mastering this important and evolving endoscopic spine technique in order to improve their patients' outcomes.

Richard G. Ellenbogen, MD, FACS
Theodore S. Roberts Professor and Chair
Department of Neurological Surgery
University of Washington
Seattle, Washington

Foreword

It is with great pleasure that I accept the invitation to write a foreword to Professor Hofstetter's wonderfully organized and executed *Atlas of Full-Endoscopic Spine Surgery*. As surgeons dedicated to the careful diagnosis and treatment of spinal pathology, our ultimate goal is to deliver the highest quality of care in order to achieve the best possible outcomes for our patients.

Unquestionably, the evolution of spinal surgery has rapidly progressed in recent decades.

As a consequence, we as surgeons, are constantly exposed to new technologies and have to ask ourselves difficult questions that sometimes do not have clear answers:

• Is this new technology really going to improve my ability to take care of patients?

• Is this here to stay or is this just a temporary trend that will fail to deliver the results promised and ultimately fade?

• Was this technology born out of a true surgical need or is it pushed for other reasons, such as industry-interest or by surgeons' egos?

• Finally, am I at a stage in my career where I can/should invest time and resources in learning this skill, and if so, how can I best do this without compromising patient safety and care?

These are certainly the questions I ask myself as I wander through the halls of our many meetings or peruse the spinal journals that land on my desk on a daily basis. I marvel at the display of technical gadgets from navigation and robotic technology, the wonders of biological disc regeneration, minimally invasive surgery, and the latest implant designs that promise higher fusion rates or faster patient recovery. Fortunately, Professor Hofstetter and co-authors finally give us some clear guidance in the area of spinal endoscopy.

Spinal endoscopy, which has transformed in recent years, certainly falls into the category of techniques that fascinate but also intimidate us spine surgeons: Did you ever find yourself watching a video clip of endoscopic spinal surgery at a meeting, or glance at articles and manuscripts describing endoscopic procedures and feeling completely lost, confused, and wondering if your understanding of the spinal anatomy is just not sophisticated enough to follow along? Do you get irritated when you overhear surgeons using many different (usually company coined) terms describing a particular surgery and it turns out they are all referring to the same procedure?

Well, this book will help you understand! It hits exactly the right spot; it is short, concise, and comprehensively written in understandable language. It is edited and written by experts in the field who went through a learning curve that we as spine surgeons who were trained in open or more "traditional" MIS surgery (mainly tubular or specular) can understand and potentially replicate. Professor Hofstetter picked up endoscopy as a natural extension after he understood and mastered "tubology." He came from where most of us are right now. And this is exactly where the strength of this book is.

Did you wonder how endoscopic surgeons create a working space in a tight spinal canal in the presence of severe stenosis? Go to Chapter 9.1 and you find a detailed description that is practical, easy to understand, and well-illustrated! One of the most satisfying procedures in my practice is the unilateral tubular approach for bilateral decompression for lumbar spinal stenosis. Chapter 14 shows a clear and understandable pathway for achieving similar decompression via the endoscope. The "Pearls and Pitfalls" that are integrated into most chapters are my favorites and provide valuable advice.

In short, this is a book that we were looking for. It is time to accept that endoscopic surgery is here to stay and will eventually replace and/or enhance many procedures that we do as open or "traditional" MIS surgeries in our daily practice. There is no doubt that spinal endoscopy will help us come closer to our ultimate goal of delivering the highest possible quality of care and achieving the best possible outcomes for our patients.

Roger Härtl, MD
Professor of Neurological Surgery
Director of Spinal Surgery
Director, Weill Cornell Medicine Center
for Comprehensive Spine Care
New York, New York

Preface

Recent advances in spine surgery have been nothing short of breathtaking. Full-endoscopic spine surgery is an emerging technique which has had a dramatic impact on the worldwide practice of spine surgery. Despite the rapid evolution of endoscopic spine surgery in past few years, there has been a relative lack of consistency in nomenclature, operative technique, and surgical goals within the global spine community. The resulting differences have stymied true academic discussion on the role full-endoscopic spine surgery plays in the treatment of spinal pathology.

This book is intended to describe the standard surgical technique of full-endoscopic spine surgery and its nuances to residents, fellows, and spine surgeons, who are interested in performing these procedures. This book is designed in the form of an atlas but also serves as a textbook. We consider this layout ideal, since the spine surgeon learns relevant anatomy and endoscope-specific technical vignettes by studying the images. This book also provides insights into the appropriate indications and surgical techniques in a step-by-step fashion, including special cases and strategies to manage intraoperative complications.

The book is organized into the following three sections: basic tenets, step-by-step description of common approaches, and special cases and challenges. Critical surgical concepts required to carry out full-endoscopic spine surgery are discussed in a detailed manner.

The first section highlights relevant spinal anatomy that is needed to efficiently and safely perform full-endoscopic spine surgery. In addition, this section contains a detailed description of endoscopic technology and provides information about special instruments that are used in endoscopic spine surgery. Finally, we include a description of common endoscopic tasks which greatly enhance and promote teaching of these surgical techniques.

The second section describes full-endoscopic spine procedures in a step-by-step fashion and sheds light on the common mistakes and pitfalls to avoid.

In contrast to traditional open spine surgery, the dynamic and small visual field of endoscopic spine surgery requires the spine surgeon to be vigilant regarding small details to help provide full orientation to locational anatomy. A critical element of endoscopic spine surgery is the precision of the approach; the surgeon is required to marry preoperative planning, intraoperative imaging, and controlled dissection to quickly dock onto a well-defined anatomic area. A major part of the learning curve involves mastering this transition. We therefore identified optimal *target areas* for all endoscopic procedures. The target areas are easily discernable on fluoroscopic imaging, have unam-biguous tactile properties, and allow for quick transition to visualization once the endoscope is in place. Importantly, the target areas have anatomical features, making them identifiable within the very limited field of view provided by endoscopic spine surgery. This is necessary since full-endoscopic spine surgery does not afford the luxury of exposing multiple anatomical structures that can be utilized in concert, as is the case during traditional spine surgery. The step-by-step description has been developed during the extensive teaching experience of the editors. This section also introduces the classical surgical concept of *principal anatomical landmarks* to full endoscopic spine surgery. Principal anatomical landmarks are highly reliable bony landmarks that allow for safe identification of neural structures. If utilized appropriately, they also allow for visual confirmation of complete neural decompression upon completion of full-endoscopic spine procedures, which has long been a major criticism of these procedures.

The third section describes the common modifications required and special tasks performed to manage special cases or complications, including dural lacerations or intraoperative bleeding.

The mission of this book is to provide a framework of the endoscopic surgical technique and also help contextualize the role of full-endoscopic spine surgery in the treatment of spinal pathology. We utilize the recently introduced worldwide AOSpine nomenclature, and a similar step-by-step curriculum of these procedures will be utilized in practical courses. Eventually, standardization will allow for more productive exchanges of ideas, further evolution of surgical techniques, and will hopefully lay the groundwork for a combined effort to better investigate patient outcomes following these procedures.

We believe that full-endoscopic spine surgery will prove to be a great asset in the light of current clinical challenges, including an aging patient population, increased medical comorbidities, and elevated expectations regarding postoperative pain and recovery. However, while we strongly believe that full-endoscopic spine surgery constitutes a crucial part of the armamentarium for the complex spine surgeon, it cannot replace traditional spine surgery. Severe spinal deformity, mechanical instability, and trauma have well established surgical remedies which cannot, currently, be replaced by full-endoscopic spine surgery. While we expect the borders between traditional, minimally invasive, and full-endoscopic techniques to be in flux, a complex spine surgeon should have insight into all of these procedures in order to choose the most sensitive option for a given pathology in each individual patient. It is paramount for the global spine surgery community to participate in an academic dialogue to elucidate the proper indications for full-endoscopic spine surgery.

Following the framework of this book and the structured step-by-step instructions will therefore necessarily be a great asset to any spine surgeon who wishes to leverage technological advancements to elevate the quality of care they provide to their patients. We have witnessed an unprecedented enthusiasm among many spine surgeons, both novice and seasoned, once they experienced the impact that this novel technology has on patient care. We hope that this book will serve as a foundation to establish, develop, and teach full-endoscopic spine surgery to the next generation of spine surgeons.

Christoph P. Hofstetter, MD, PhD, FACS
Sebastian Ruetten, MD
Yue Zhou, MD, PhD
Michael Y. Wang, MD, FACS

Contributors

G. Gamian Brusko, MD
Resident
Department of Neurosurgery
University of Miami
Miami, Florida

Daniel Carr, DO
Attending Spine Surgeon
Michigan Spine and Brain Surgeons
Southfield, Michigan

J. N. Alastair Gibson, DSc, FRCSEd
Attending Spine Surgeon
Spire Murrayfield Hospital
Edinburgh, UK

Saqib Hasan, MD
Attending Spine Surgeon
Webster Orthopedics Spine Institute
Oakland, California

Christoph P. Hofstetter, MD, PhD, FACS
Associate Professor
Department of Neurological Surgery
University of Washington Medical Center
Seattle, Washington

Jun Ho Lee, MD, PhD
Associate Professor
Department of Neurosurgery
Kyung Hee University Medical Center
Seoul, Republic of Korea

Lynn McGrath, MD
Resident
Department of Neurological Surgery
University of Washington
Seattle, Washington

Sebastian Ruetten, MD
Attending Spine Surgeon
Center for Spine Surgery and Pain Therapy
Center for Orthopaedics and Traumatology of the
    St. Elisabeth Group – Catholic Hospital Rhein-Ruhr
St. Anna Hospital Herne/Marien Hospital Herne University
    Hospital/Marien Hospital Witten
Herne, Germany

Ralf Wagner, MD
Attending Spine Surgeon
Ligamenta Spine Center
Frankfurt, Germany

Michael Y. Wang, MD, FACS
Professor
Departments of Neurosurgery and Rehab Medicine
University of Miami School of Medicine
Miami, Florida

Yue Zhou, MD, PhD
Professor
Department of Orthopaedics
Xinqiao Hospital
Army Medical University
Chongqing, China

Part 1

Introduction

1 Anesthesia and Rapid Recovery

G. Gamian Brusko and Michael Y. Wang

1.1 Introduction

Full-endoscopic spine surgery is an ultraminimally invasive surgical technique that affords the spine surgeon an opportunity to utilize anesthetic methods other than general anesthesia. Because endoscopic surgery focuses on minimizing surgical morbidity, anesthetic protocols that reduce the associated risks of sedation should be employed to complement the endoscopic surgical approach. This chapter will provide a brief introduction to the aims of rapid recovery, discuss the important principles as they apply to spine surgery, and outline anesthetic protocols for use during endoscopic procedures.

1.2 General Principles of Rapid Recovery

Rapid recovery or "fast-track" surgery protocols are designed to reduce the morbidity associated with surgery and shorten the length of hospital stay following a surgical procedure. Also referred to as enhanced recovery after surgery (ERAS), such pathways focus on optimizing patients for surgery preoperatively, reducing surgical stress intraoperatively, and improving pain control postoperatively. Henrik Kehlet, a Danish colorectal surgeon, was the first to describe these principles of enhanced recovery in an organized fashion, which focus on minimizing the surgical stress response and preventing complications related to anesthesia, surgical technique, and postoperative hospitalization.[1] Importantly, Kehlet described ERAS as a multidisciplinary approach for enhancing patient care. Thus, anesthetic principles play an important role perioperatively in rapid recovery.

1.3 Key Components

Of the many important perioperative interventions in an ERAS protocol, there are four key elements in which anesthesia should play a critical role: (1) preoperative medication optimization, (2) intraoperative conscious sedation, (3) local injectable anesthetics, and (4) postoperative multimodal analgesic regimens. Each of these interventions will be briefly discussed to create a foundation in rapid recovery techniques for the endoscopic spine surgeon and are summarized in ▶ Table 1.1.

Prior to any surgical procedure, several steps are taken to optimize patients for surgery. Managing comorbidities, promoting regular exercise, and improving nutritional status preoperatively are well known to improve outcomes. In addition to these recommendations, rapid recovery pathways also optimize medications before surgery, focusing primarily on pain medications, which is of importance in patients undergoing spine surgery. As some patients suffer from chronic pain related to their spinal disease, understanding the role of non-narcotic pharmacotherapy options is critical. This may limit the amount of narcotic medications consumed, which has been shown to improve outcomes for spine patients. Most notably, the preoperative administration of gabapentinoids (pregabalin or gabapentin) reduces postoperative pain, total morphine consumption, and morphine-related complications such as nausea following spine surgery.[2] Additionally, preemptive multimodal analgesic regimens that include celecoxib, pregabalin, extended-release oxycodone, and acetaminophen prior to surgery have been successfully employed in spine surgery for decreasing postoperative pain.[3] For patients undergoing decompressive surgery, anti-inflammatory medications are a useful adjuvant. There is also an emerging body of evidence that for short segment fusions the use of these medications is unlikely to reduce the arthrodesis rate. Managing patients' narcotic usage prior to surgery may temper their opioid requirements after surgery and facilitate both decreased pain and a shorter hospital stay.

Full-endoscopic spine surgery also provides a unique opportunity to utilize conscious sedation within a rapid recovery pathway. While commonly employed for minor surgical procedures, conscious sedation with ketamine and propofol has recently been used for endoscopic spine surgery.[4] Importantly, the addition of ketamine to the sedation protocol decreases the postoperative opioid requirement in spine patients. Furthermore, the use of total intravenous (IV) anesthesia has also been shown to reduce the incidence of postoperative nausea and vomiting as part of a conscious sedation protocol.[5] Obviating the need for general anesthesia promotes a faster recovery from sedation and therefore enables early mobilization within a few hours after surgery.

A further advantage of conscious sedation is the neurological feedback from the patient. Endoscopic spine surgery is frequently performed in an outpatient setting where electrophysiologic neuromonitoring may be impractical from a resource or economic perspective. As such, the ability of the patient to

Table 1.1 Key anesthesia-related interventions in a rapid recovery pathway for endoscopic spine surgery

Preoperative	
• Medication optimization • Preparation of the patient	Use of gabapentinoids and/or preemptive multimodal analgesic regimens Educational programs and prehabilitation with physical therapy
Intraoperative	
• Conscious sedation	Intravenous ketamine and propofol to maintain light to moderate sedation
• Local injectable anesthetics	Long-acting local anesthetics at the very limited areas of soft-tissue trauma
Postoperative	
• Multimodal analgesia • Rapid mobilization	Use of opioid-sparing medications to limit narcotic consumption and its side effects Prevention of complications from prolonged bed rest and rapid discharge to home

report nerve irritation can be helpful for preventing intraoperative complications. The sensitivity of the dorsal root ganglion (DRG) to trauma has also led some endoscopic surgeons to be wary of false-negative reports from intraoperative monitoring. In that setting, a sedated but responsive patient is more likely to detect proximity, traction, or trauma to the DRG.

The third key intraoperative component of enhanced recovery is wound infiltration with local anesthetics, which improves analgesia and lessens the need for narcotic medications after surgery. Bupivacaine has traditionally been used for this purpose. Ropivacaine has a similarly long half-life and has the added advantage of reduced cardiotoxicity. However, a newer formulation that increases the analgesic period has demonstrated even greater efficacy in spine surgery. Liposomal bupivacaine provides up to 72 hours of local analgesic relief and can be injected directly along the pedicle screw tracts when placing percutaneous screws in endoscopic spine surgery. For minimally invasive fusions, use of liposomal bupivacaine has demonstrated reductions in length of stay, pain scores, and narcotic consumption.[6] Although more costly than standard bupivacaine, incorporation of liposomal bupivacaine into a rapid recovery surgical pathway has reduced acute care costs by several thousand dollars per patient, greatly exceeding the medication expense.[7]

The goals of anesthesia in the postoperative period are similar for any procedure, but also allow a large percentage of patients to be treated in the outpatient setting. Measures to provide adequate pain relief and to limit common complications and side effects such as respiratory depression or nausea and vomiting should be employed. To achieve these aims in a rapid recovery pathway, however, a multimodal analgesic regimen is often utilized. Combinations of various opioid-sparing medications including acetaminophen, nonsteroidal anti-inflammatory diseases (NSAIDs), gabapentin, S-ketamine, dexamethasone, and ondansetron have shown a benefit in reducing pain and nausea postoperatively.[8] The use of locally injected anesthetics discussed earlier, as well as immediate postoperative infusion of 1 g of IV acetaminophen may also be used within a multimodal regimen.

An important way in which these interventions enhance patient recovery is hastening patients' time to ambulation after surgery. The use of conscious sedation and non-narcotic postoperative pain management allows patients to awaken faster and in less pain. This enables early and aggressive mobilization of patients with the nursing staff and physical therapy, which has demonstrated a clear benefit for shortening hospital stays.

1.4 Anesthesia Protocol

Based on rapid recovery principles, we have previously designed an enhanced recovery pathway to complement a transforaminal endoscopic lumbar interbody fusion (see Chapter 17).[9] More recently, we have expanded on the initial iteration to incorporate the interventions described in this chapter. Here we outline a simple protocol that the endoscopic spine surgeon may follow for inclusion in their practice.

On the day of surgery, patients are administered 300 mg of oral gabapentin in addition to the traditional preanesthesia medications. Once the patient is properly positioned for

Table 1.2 Outline of rapid recovery protocol for endoscopic spine surgery

Preoperative
• Addition of gabapentin to the preanesthetic medication regimen

Intraoperative
• Conscious sedation with IV ketamine and propofol
• Injection of liposomal bupivacaine dilution along pedicle screw tracts
• Use of endoscopic visualization to minimize soft-tissue trauma

Postoperative
• Immediate intravenous (IV) infusion of acetaminophen
• Oral acetaminophen-oxycodone and IV hydromorphone as needed for severe pain
• Encourage early mobilization

surgery, supplemental oxygen via face mask or nasal cannula is provided. Close monitoring by the anesthesiologist is required due to the lack of intubation. Ketamine and propofol are then continuously infused to maintain light to moderate sedation, which allows for feedback from the patient if the surgeon contacts neural structures. Injection of a 1:2 dilution of 20 mL of liposomal bupivacaine along the pedicle screw tracts is completed immediately prior to screw insertion. No narcotic, spinal, or epidural anesthesia is used. Immediately following the conclusion of the procedure, IV infusion of 1 g of acetaminophen is begun while the patient remains in the operating room. Postoperatively, patients are given oral acetaminophen-oxycodone and IV hydromorphone as needed for pain, and they should be encouraged to mobilize as early as possible. While most patients require some narcotics, the amount consumed is significantly reduced compared to a traditional analgesic regimen. Complications such as nausea, dysphagia, and memory loss also occur less frequently. A summary of these interventions is provided in ▶ Table 1.2.

1.5 Summary

This chapter has provided a brief introduction to the aims of rapid recovery and how certain anesthetic interventions can be applied to endoscopic spine surgery perioperatively. Various techniques and management options are available to create a foundation of enhanced recovery upon which the spine surgeon can increase their expertise. The subspecialty of full-endoscopic spine surgery lends itself well to the principles of rapid recovery.

References

[1] Kehlet H. Multimodal approach to control postoperative pathophysiology and rehabilitation. Br J Anaesth. 1997; 78(5):606–617
[2] Liu B, Liu R, Wang L. A meta-analysis of the preoperative use of gabapentinoids for the treatment of acute postoperative pain following spinal surgery. Medicine (Baltimore). 2017; 96(37):e8031
[3] Kim SI, Ha KY, Oh IS. Preemptive multimodal analgesia for postoperative pain management after lumbar fusion surgery: a randomized controlled trial. Eur Spine J. 2016; 25(5):1614–1619
[4] Wang MY, Grossman J. Endoscopic minimally invasive transforaminal interbody fusion without general anesthesia: initial clinical experience with 1-year follow-up. Neurosurg Focus. 2016; 40(2):E13

[5] Peng K, Liu H-Y, Liu S-L, Ji F-H. Dexmedetomidine-fentanyl compared with midazolam-fentanyl for conscious sedation in patients undergoing lumbar disc surgery. Clin Ther. 2016; 38(1):192–201.e2

[6] Kim J, Burke SM, Kryzanski JT, et al. The role of liposomal bupivacaine in reduction of postoperative pain after transforaminal lumbar interbody fusion: a clinical study. World Neurosurg. 2016; 91:460–467

[7] Wang MY, Chang HK, Grossman J. Reduced acute care costs with the ERAS(R) minimally invasive transforaminal lumbar interbody fusion compared with conventional minimally invasive transforaminal lumbar interbody fusion. Neurosurgery. 2016; 83(4):827–834

[8] Mathiesen O, Dahl B, Thomsen BA, et al. A comprehensive multimodal pain treatment reduces opioid consumption after multilevel spine surgery. Eur Spine J. 2013; 22(9):2089–2096

[9] Wang MY, Chang PY, Grossman J. Development of an enhanced recovery after surgery (ERAS) approach for lumbar spinal fusion. J Neurosurg Spine. 2017; 26(4):411–418

2 Radiation Safety in Full-Endoscopic Spine Surgery

Lynn McGrath and Christoph P. Hofstetter

2.1 Introduction

Minimally invasive approaches to the spine require intraoperative imaging techniques that allow for visualization of the bony spinal anatomy without the need for physical exposure of the target structures. While the use of two-dimensional fluoroscopy or portable intraoperative computed tomography (CT) is increasing, the C-arm image intensifier fluoroscope remains prevalent and the primary source of radiation exposure in most operating rooms. The C-arm is comprised of a mobile X-ray source that is located at one end of a C-shaped arm and aimed at an X-ray detector or image intensifier located at the other end (▶ Fig. 2.1). The X-ray source is usually housed within a cone that serves to maintain a minimum safe distance to the patient. This source generates X-rays that penetrate a patient's soft tissues and are subsequently detected by the image intensifier. The image intensifier converts these X-rays into visible light, allowing interpretation by the surgeon. The C-arm is generally able to be move horizontally, vertically, or swivel on its axis, enabling images of a patient's anatomy from almost any angle. The ability to provide flexible real-time imaging of relevant anatomy is the biggest advantage of the C-arm fluoroscope, and as a result it is the most common modality for intraoperative spine imaging in the United States. Thus, familiarity with radiographic techniques is fundamental to the ability of a spine surgeon to successfully adopt and implement minimally invasive approaches into their practice. The intimate relationship and physical proximity of pathology with sensitive neural and stabilizing osseoligamentous structures necessitate a high degree of radiographic precision throughout the duration of surgery.

2.2 Occupational Radiation Guidelines

The vast majority of intraoperative imaging modalities leverage property of X-rays to penetrate soft tissues and delineate bony anatomy. Radiography, fluoroscopy, and CT all produce ionizing radiation, which in certain dosages can become detrimental to human health. Medical professionals are considered radiation workers by the U.S. Occupational Safety and Health Administration (OSHA) and are advised to adhere to exposure guidelines put forth by the National Council on Radiation Protection and Measurements (NCRP) and the International Commission on Radiological Protection (ICRP). Radiation workers can quantify and track their occupational exposure to the ionizing radiation generated by medical devices using specialized units of measurement. The sievert (Sv) is one such unit and is defined as 1 J/kg of body tissue, averaged over the whole body. It is the preferred unit when considering the risk to patients and health professionals in a clinical setting. In occupational settings, radiation exposure is measured in millisieverts (mSv), or 1/1,000 Sv. The maximum exposure limit delineated by the NCRP and ICRP is 50 mSv/y (▶ Table 2.1) For context, the average effective dose of radiation delivered to each person in the United States is 6.2 mSv.[1] The majority of this exposure comes from natural background radiation in the form of household accumulation of radon and thoron gases (~2.8 mSv), cosmic radiation (0.3 mSv), and medical procedures such as CT (10 mSv for a full-body CT).

Occupational radiation exposure is tightly regulated because there is essentially no dose of radiation that is considered risk free. Human studies have demonstrated a roughly linear relationship between radiation exposure and cancer risk, and while

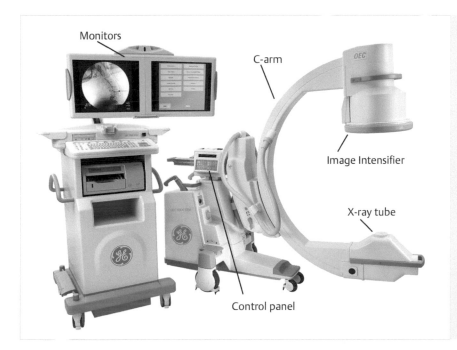

Fig. 2.1 Components of an intraoperative C-arm.

Monitors

C-arm

Image Intensifier

X-ray tube

Control panel

Table 2.1 National Council on Radiation Protection and Measurements effective dose limits for occupational workers

Occupational exposure	Dose/S.I.
Effective dose equivalent limits for stochastic effects	Annual: 50 mSv (cumulative 10 mSv × age in y)
Equivalent annual dose to tissue's nonstochastic effects	
Lens of eye	150 mSv
Skin, hand, and feet	500 mSv

a single exposure event of 100 mSv is known to increase the risk of certain cancers in human, the risks of radiation exposure are in fact cumulative over a lifetime.

2.3 Radiation Safety

Radiation workers in health care have been well documented to exhibit the effects of ionizing radiation. General orthopaedic surgeons develop tumors at a fivefold increased rate when compared with other hospital staff presumably due to disproportionate levels of radiation exposure. Spine surgeons are exposed to particularly high doses of radiation as C-arm free hand fluoroscopy-guided pedicle screw placement has been shown to generate 10 to 12 times the radiation exposure compared to navigated technique.[2] Cancer risk may be the most concerning but is certainly not the only health risk associated with occupational radiation exposure. Radiation workers have been shown to develop cataracts at 4.6 times the rate of nonradiation workers.

2.4 ALARA (As Low As Reasonably Achievable) Principle

2.4.1 Restrict the Area and Duration of Exposure

Before obtaining fluoroscopic images, the C-arm position and setup should be optimized in order to reduce the number of redundant off-target images. Laser guides should be used to move the C-arm to the anatomical area of question. The image intensifier should be paced to the skin as close as possible, which in combination with tight collimation of the fluoroscopic beam helps increase the efficiency of image capture. Life fluoroscopy should be avoided and pulsed fluoroscopic images obtained. The later technique decreases the radiation exposure by up to 30%. As high-quality images are often unnecessary and lead to needless radiation exposure, lower quality images should be a surgeon's default with the use of high-quality images reserved for a challenging or essential views (► Fig. 2.2). In conclusion, efficient use of fluoroscopy should be considered a surgical skill to be honed like any other.

2.4.2 Get as Much Distance to the Radiation Source as Achievable

When performing fluoroscopy, radiation exposure is significantly lower on the side of the image intensifier than on the side of the source. Thus, the surgeon should make an effort to stand away from the source whenever possible. During cross-table imaging, the surgeon should attempt to stand on the side of the image intensifier (► Fig. 2.3). When performing through-table imaging, the radiation source should be placed under the patient with the image intensifier as close to the top of the patient as possible. The surgeon should avoid sitting but stand in order to decrease the exposure of the eyes (► Fig. 2.3). Most of the radiation emitted by a C-arm that reaches the surgeon and surgical team members originates from backscatter and decreases as a function of distance. The exposure is inversely proportional to the square of the distance from the source. As a rule of thumb, standing away 2 m from the radiation source reduces dose to negligible levels.

2.4.3 Protect Yourself against Radiation Exposure

Adequate protective equipment is essential and should be used by the surgical team and anesthesia in every case during which fluoroscopy is anticipated. Leaded vests, skirts, and thyroid

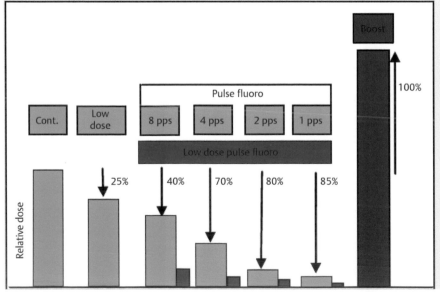

Fig. 2.2 Effect of various C-arm settings on the relative dose. Note the dramatic reduction in relative dose by using the pulsed fluoroscopy setting. The reduction is further enhanced by using the low-dose setting. The boost function on the contrary greatly increases the relative dose emitted by the C-arm.

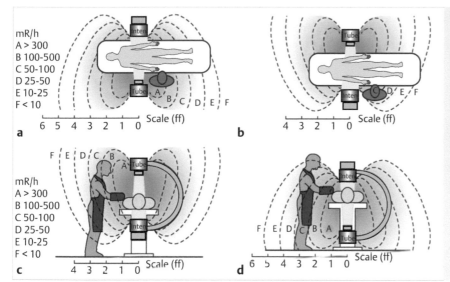

mR/h
A > 300
B 100-500
C 50-100
D 25-50
E 10-25
F < 10

Scale (ff)

a

b

mR/h
A > 300
B 100-500
C 50-100
D 25-50
E 10-25
F < 10

Scale (ff)

c

d

Fig. 2.3 Impact of C-arm positioning on surgeon exposure during cross-table and anteroposterior (AP) fluoroscopy. **(a)** During cross-table examination with the X-ray tube on the side of the surgeon, the exposure may be greater than 300 mR/h. **(b)** Turning the C-arm, dramatically decreases the exposure. **(c)** During AP fluoroscopy, the surgeon is exposed to high doses with the X-ray tube above the patient. **(d)** Turning the C-arm dramatically decreases the exposure of the surgeon. Note that if the surgeon stands upright, scattered radiation to the face may be one-fourth as great compared to when the surgeon is leaning down toward the patient.

shields are the standard and should be rated to at least 0.5-mm lead equivalents. Vests with sleeves, skullcaps, and other additional forms of protection have become available and are beginning to see widespread adoption. Leaded safety glasses should be worn during every case in which fluoroscopy is anticipated. Leaded glasses are essential in the prevention of cataract formation and should be rated to at least 0.75-mm lead equivalents. These essential pieces of personal protective equipment should be formally tested on a regular basis to ensure their continued efficacy.

2.5 Emerging Technologies

In order to minimize radiation exposure to both the surgical team and patient, spine surgeons are beginning to transition away from fluoroscopy and toward other imaging modalities that provide intraoperative CT or CT-like images. These techniques can provide either two-dimensional fluoroscopic images like a conventional C-arm or cross-sectional imaging in multiple planes by taking many fluoroscopic shots circumferentially around a patient. These cross-sectional images are useful for surgeons in evaluating screw trajectories, pedicle breaches, and deformity correction. These image sets can also be used as reference images in conjunction with surgical navigation technology allowing surgeons to use image-guided equipment. Despite the high cost and complexity of the equipment, image-

guided surgery has the potential to substantially reduce the amount of radiation exposure to surgeons and surgical staff and increase the accuracy with which hardware is placed.

2.6 Conclusion

Understanding imaging technology and radiation safety is an essential skillset for the surgeon to master like any other component of surgery. Efficient use of current modalities will keep patients and surgical staff safe and help maintain a high degree of surgical precision. Advances in intraoperative imaging techniques and image-guided surgery are expensive and complex but have the potential to increase precision while decreasing radiation exposure. A high degree of familiarity with these modalities will further empower any surgeon practicing minimally invasive surgical (MIS) or endoscopic spine surgical techniques.

References

[1] NCRP. NCRP Report No. 160, Ionizing Radiation Exposure of the Population of the United States. 2006. Available at: https://ncrponline.org/publications/reports/ncrp-report-160-2/

[2] Villard J, Ryang YM, Demetriades AK, et al. Radiation exposure to the surgeon and the patient during posterior lumbar spinal instrumentation: a prospective randomized comparison of navigated versus non-navigated freehand techniques. Spine. 2014; 39(13):1004–1009

3 Essential Imaging in Full-Endoscopic Spine Surgery

Daniel Carr and Christoph P. Hofstetter

3.1 Introduction

The successful and efficient adoption of full-endoscopic spine surgery requires the surgeon to be an expert in obtaining and interpreting high-quality intraoperative fluoroscopic images. The extremely minimal access nature of full-endoscopic technique necessitates precise fluoroscopic localization of target areas to allow for preoperative determination optimal starting points and trajectories. During the procedure, radiographically determined anatomic landmarks serve as the foundation for efficient surgical flow and safe identification of neural elements.

3.2 Features of Intraoperative Fluoroscopy

Fluoroscopic images are associated with certain well-known radiographic phenomena that must be anticipated and mitigated in order to safely and effectively utilize the modality for intraoperative imaging. If well understood, these properties can be leveraged by the surgeon to enhance visualization of target anatomy and pathology.

3.2.1 Magnification

The X-ray beam is emitted by the X-ray tube and travels through tissue to the X-ray image intensifier. As this detector has a much larger surface area than the point from which the photons are originally emitted, the beam must diverge as it passes through air and tissue in order to eventually fill the entirety of the detector plate. This divergence causes imaged anatomic structures to appear larger than they are in reality. This effect is more pronounced the closer the tissue is relative to the X-ray tube and this reliable effect can be leveraged by the

surgeon to craft an image with characteristics specific to their current need. For example, if the surgeon desires a wide field of view for localization or to examine the entirety of a construct they may move the spine further away from the X-ray tube to visualize multiple vertebral segments. If they wish to magnify a specific segment of the spine or particular structure, the X-ray tube may be moved closer to the patient for an image portraying anatomy with a higher level of detail.

3.2.2 Distortion

The image intensifier has a curved input surface that consists of an input phosphor (converts X-rays into optical photons) and a photocathode (converts optical photons into photoelectrons). The curvature of the input surface causes a more severe distortion and greater distance between equidistant points at the periphery of the image compared to the center (► Fig. 3.1 **a**). A large field of view enhances the distortion, where the curvature of the input phosphor surface is the greatest at the edges of the image. Modern flat panel image receptors are generally free from image distortion.

3.2.3 Parallax

As with magnification, this phenomenon derives from the divergence of photons within the X-ray beam as they travel from the emitter to the detector. This divergence is most significant at the periphery of the beam or at the margins of the image produced. The result is that structures at the center of an image are most accurately depicted, while peripheral structures will be projected slightly distorted. The region of interest should always be placed at the center of the image to avoid misinterpretation (► Fig. 3.1 **b**).

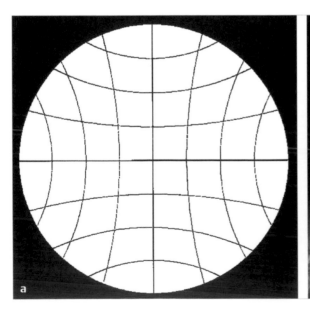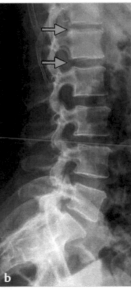

Fig. 3.1 Artifacts in fluoroscopic imaging. **(a)** Schematic illustrates the distortion artifact most pronounced in the periphery of the field of view. **(b)** Illustration of parallax on a lateral lumbar X-ray. Parallax lead to the appearance of narrowed T11–T12 and T12–L1 disk spaces *(green arrows)*.

3.3 Fundamental Fluoroscopic Images for Full-Endoscopic Spine Surgery

3.3.1 Lumbar Spine

The most essential radiographic images for lumbar endoscopic spine surgery are a true anteroposterior (AP) and lateral view of the vertebral body of the index level. Most subsequent imaging and targeting depends on these images. A proper AP image of the lumbar spine should demonstrate the spinous process equidistant from the pedicles bilaterally. Pedicles are seen in the upper half of the vertebral body perfectly aligned. The vertebral body endplates should align perfectly and should produce a single endplate shadow when properly superimposed (▶ Fig. 3.2 **a**).

The other fundamental view of the lumbar spine is a true lateral view. A proper lateral image of the spine should demonstrate superimposed pedicles and perfectly aligned endplates at the index level (▶ Fig. 3.2 **b**). The posterior wall of the vertebral body should be parallel to the X-ray beam. Facet joints should be seen with the superior articular process (SAP) clearly discernable.

3.3.2 Interlaminar Technique

When performing an interlaminar endoscopic lumbar approach, the first step is a perfect AP endplate view of the caudal index level (▶ Fig. 3.3 **a**). The endplate view serves as the baseline for determining an optimal rostrocaudal approach angle. Addition of approximately 0 to 5 degrees of distal C-arm tilt is typically required in the upper lumbar segments and

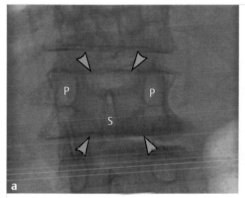
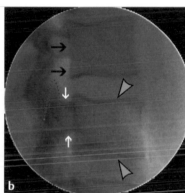

Fig. 3.2 Fundamental lumbar spine X-rays.
(a) Anteroposterior endplate view of the lumbar spine. The endplates (*green arrowheads*) are parallel and produce single endplate shadows. The spinous process (S) is equidistant to the pedicles bilaterally. Pedicles (P) are seen in the upper half of the vertebral body. **(b)** A true lateral X-ray of the lumbar spine. The endplates (*green arrowheads*) produce single endplate shadows. The posterior walls of the vertebral bodies are parallel to the beam (*black arrows*) and pedicles are superimposed (*white arrows*). The facet joint is seen and the superior articular process (*red dotted line*) is clearly discernable.

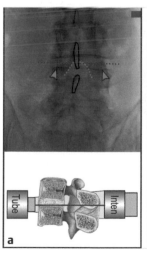
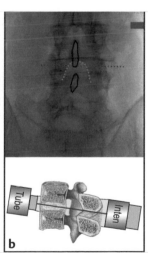
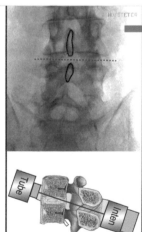

Fig. 3.3 Adjustment of the C-arm for the interlaminar approach. **(a)** First an anteroposterior endplate view of the superior endplate of the caudal index level is obtained (L3/L4; *green arrowheads*). The *red dotted line* indicates the center of the index level disc. **(b)** The addition of distal tilt to the rostrocaudal X-ray beam angle moves the projection of the superior spinous process space rostrally. **(c)** Once the gap between spinous processes is centered over the projection of the disk space an ideal rostrocaudal trajectory has been determined. Note the inferomedial edge of the rostral index lamina (*green dotted line*) that serves as a target area for the interlaminar approach.

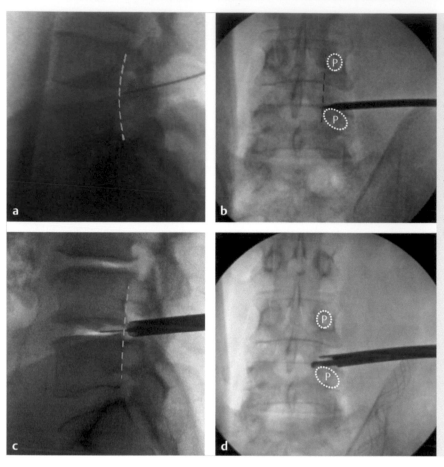

Fig. 3.4 Important radiographic structures for the transforaminal approach. (a) The spinal needle is advanced along the ventrolateral aspect of the superior articular process (*red dotted line*). Of note, the tip of the needle should remain posterior to the posterior vertebral line (*green dotted line*). (b) The medial pedicle line (*blue dotted line*) connects the most medial aspects of the index level pedicles (P). This line indicates the lateral aspect of the neural elements.
(c) Maintaining the tip of the tubular retractor dorsal to the posterior vertebral line facilitates visualization of the neural elements. (d) The Kerrison rongeur may be placed onto the caudal index level pedicle to radiographically confirm this principal anatomical landmark of the transforaminal approach.

addition of approximately 10 to 15 degrees in the lower lumbar segments. The goal is to center the spinous processes over the projection of the disk space (▸ Fig. 3.3 **b**). This technique provides a starting point and approach trajectory that allows for efficient access to the lateral recess and intervertebral disk. The AP X-ray (▸ Fig. 3.3 **c**) should also depict the inferomedial edge of the rostral index level lamina as it serves as the *target area* for almost all interlaminar approaches (exception is an L5/S1 approach with a wide interlaminar window).

3.3.3 Transforaminal Technique

When performing a transforaminal endoscopic approach, it is important to obtain high-quality AP and lateral views. On lateral fluoroscopic images, the SAP and the posterior vertebral line are utilized during targeting (▸ Fig. 3.4 **a,c**). The SAP servers as the *target area* for the trans-SAP and for most transforaminal approaches. The posterior vertebral line indicates the ventral border of the spinal canal—the tip of the tubular retractor should remain at or behind this line to allow for direct visualization of the neural elements. On AP X-rays, the medial pedicle line constitutes a surrogate for the lateral margin of the thecal sac or the traversing nerve root. The mediolateral position of trocar, bone trephines, and working sleeves should be referenced to this line to prevent damage to the neural elements (▸ Fig. 3.4 **b**). The caudal index-level pedicle serves as the

principal anatomical landmark for the transforaminal approaches and can be readily confirmed radiographically (▸ Fig. 3.4 **d**).

3.4 Thoracic Spine

When working in the thoracic spine, identification of the appropriate level is one of the most challenging issues. Preoperative images should include either full spine X-rays or CT. This is in particular important in cases of six lumbar vertebral bodies. Utilizing fluoroscopy, the correct level can be identified by counting rostrally from L5/S1, identifying the last rib at T12 or counting caudally from C7/T1. Identification of the correct level can also be facilitated by implantation of radiopaque particles into the index-level pedicle by interventional radiology or by using CT-guided navigation.

3.5 Cervical Spine

When performing the interlaminar approach in the cervical spine, the first step is to obtain perfect AP and lateral views. AP X-rays with the spinous process equidistant from the pedicles bilaterally confirm that the patient is not rotated. Good lateral X-rays allow for the visualization of the disk space and facet joints that facilitate determination of the approach angle (▸ Fig. 3.5).

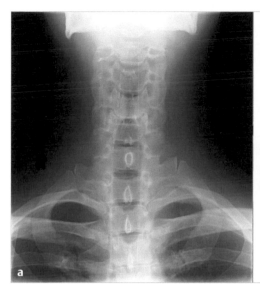 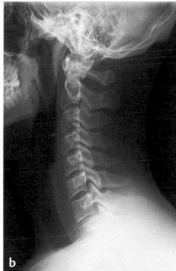

Fig. 3.5 Essential X-rays for cervical approaches. **(a)** Anteroposterior X-ray confirms that the patient is not rotated as the spinous processes are equidistant from the pedicles bilaterally. The *green dotted line* indicates the medial pedicle line. **(b)** Lateral X-ray allows for clear visualization of disk spaces (*red line*) and the facet joints (*blue line*).

3.6 Conclusion

The extremely minimal access nature of full-endoscopic spine surgery necessitates very precise radiographic visualization of target areas and bony landmarks to ensure optimal starting points, trajectories, and an effective workflow. Obtaining and interpreting high-quality intraoperative fluoroscopic images greatly facilitates full-endoscopic spinal procedures.

4 Intraoperative Navigation in Full-Endoscopic Spine Surgery

Yue Zhou

4.1 Case Example

A 47-year-old man presents with a 4-month history of right upper extremity radicular pain. The pain radiates from his neck to the right upper extremity involving the third and fourth digits. The patient rates the pain severity as 8 out of 10. On physical examination, the patient has motor weakness of his right triceps (3/5). MRI of the cervical spine reveals a right C6/C7 disk herniation (▶ Fig. 4.1 **a**). The patient underwent a *right posterior endoscopic C6/C7 foraminotomy and diskectomy assisted by intraoperative navigation*. During the surgery, a CT scan of the cervical spine was obtained and registered to the patient (▶ Fig. 4.1 **b**). Planning of the skin incision and approach trajectory were greatly facilitated by utilizing navigation (▶ Fig. 4.1 **c**). Intraoperatively, the disk sequester was seen in the axilla of the C7 nerve root and resected (▶ Fig. 4.2 **a,b**). A postoperative MRI confirmed successful removal of the disk sequester (▶ Fig. 4.2 **c**) and a CT scan suggested only minimal resection of the C6/C7 facet joint (▶ Fig. 4.2 **d**). At 1-year follow-up, the patient is neurologically intact.

4.2 Background

Full-endoscopic spine surgery is a rapidly developing surgical technique that provides surgical solutions for an increasing number of spinal ailments. Given the small surgical field of view provided by full-endoscopic spine surgery, intraoperative imaging needs to depict target areas with high accuracy in order to allow for a seamless transition from intraoperative imaging to palpation and subsequent direct visualization during the workflow. Fluoroscopic imaging is currently the standard intraoperative imaging modality for full-endoscopic spine surgery. It allows for precise intraoperative identification of various target areas (see Chapter 3). However, fluoroscopic imaging has several drawbacks. First, it exposes the surgeon and staff to high doses of radiation. Second, it only provides two-dimensional (2D) information that requires acquisition of both AP and lateral images. Finally, it does not provide continuous real-time three-dimensional (3D) information regarding the location of surgical tools. For these reasons, intraoperative navigation has been developed. Intraoperative navigation

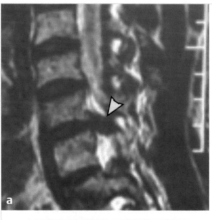
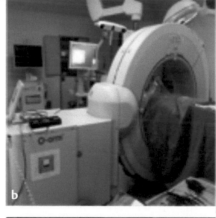
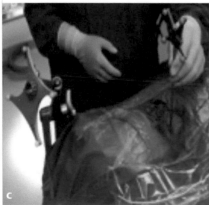
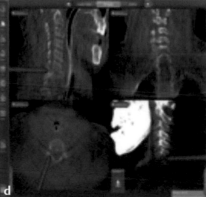

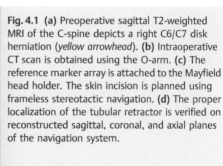

Fig. 4.1 (a) Preoperative sagittal T2-weighted MRI of the C-spine depicts a right C6/C7 disk herniation (*yellow arrowhead*). (b) Intraoperative CT scan is obtained using the O-arm. (c) The reference marker array is attached to the Mayfield head holder. The skin incision is planned using frameless stereotactic navigation. (d) The proper localization of the tubular retractor is verified on reconstructed sagittal, coronal, and axial planes of the navigation system.

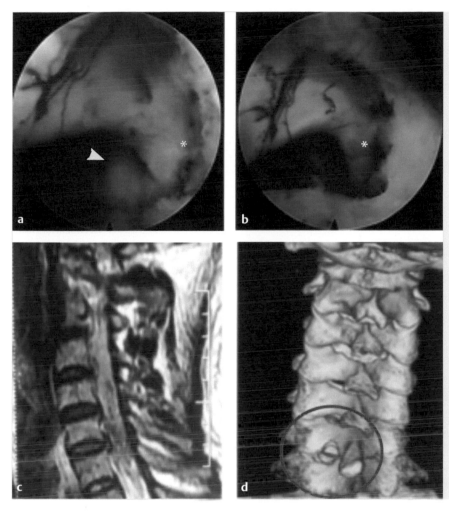

Fig. 4.2 (a) The C6/C7 disk herniation (*yellow arrowhead*) is seen in the axilla of the C7 nerve root (*asterisk*). **(b)** Intraoperative view of the decompressed C7 nerve root following diskectomy. **(c)** MRI of the C-spine after surgery confirms complete resection of the disk sequester. **(d)** Postoperative view of a 3D reconstruction depicts the limited hemilaminotomy with almost complete preservation of the facet joint.

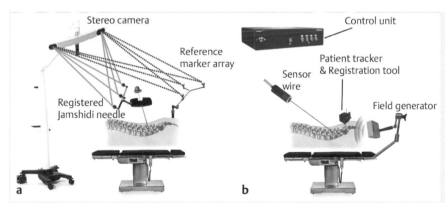

Fig. 4.3 Illustration depicting different types of navigation systems. **(a)** Optical navigation systems utilize a stereo camera that simultaneously tracks the reference marker array (*red lines*) and the registered surgical tool (*green lines*). **(b)** Electromagnetic navigation systems require a field generator that is positioned adjacent to the surgical field, a patient tracker, and a sensor wire. Note the small diameter of the sensor wire, which allows for navigation of small-diameter tools such as 18-G or Jamshidi needles.

allows the surgeon to determine the exact instrument location in 3D space in real time. There are two main types of navigation systems: optical or electromagnetic (▶ Fig. 4.3). Optical systems are most commonly used for neurosurgical and orthopaedic procedures. Optical navigation systems consist of a stereoscopic camera, a computer platform with screen, and the respective navigation software. A stereoscopic camera emits infrared light that allows determination of the position of reflective marker spheres in 3D space (Brainlab, Stealth). During the surgery, an array with marker spheres is attached to the patient's spinal column to reference the patient's spinal column in space (reference marker array). Navigated surgical instruments also carry arrays

with marker spheres to enable determination of their exact localization in reference to the spinal column (▶ Fig. 4.3 **a**). Optical systems are highly accurate and well established. Shortcomings of these systems are line-of-sight issues given that the reflective marker spheres need to be visualized by the camera. Moreover, the marker spheres are typically attached to the handle of the instruments and therefore flexible needle tips cannot be reliably navigated.

Electromagnetic fields are another strategy to allow for navigation.[1,2] A field generator is placed adjacent to the surgical field. The patient's body is registered with a tracking tool that is attached to the vertebral column. A sensor wire within the surgical tool allows determination of its location in relation to the registered spinal column (▶ Fig. 4.3 **b**). Electromagnetic navigation provides high spatial accuracy similar to optical navigation. Importantly, electromagnetic navigation is not hampered by line-of-sight restrictions inherent in optical systems and is compatible with nonrigid instruments such as puncture needles, with the potential for expanded applications in minimally invasive surgery (MIS) and percutaneous procedures where the instruments to be tracked may be flexible.[1,2] However, problems can arise with field distortion when the transmitter is moved or ferromagnetic substances approach the electromagnetic field.[3]

Importantly, intraoperative navigation has been shown to dramatically decrease radiation exposure to the surgeon and staff.[4] It has allowed us to minimize approaches in neurosurgery, to preserve function, and to improve outcomes.[5] Navigation has greatly enhanced the efficiency and accuracy of implants in both spinal procedures and orthopaedic joint replacements.[6] In 2018, the Department of Orthopaedics at the Xinqiao Hospital (The Third Military Medical University) introduced a visualized endoscopic electromagnetic navigation system (SEEssys, joimax-China, Fiagon, Germany). It enables tracking of surgical instruments in 3D space, which allows surgeons to navigate the spinal anatomy using a preoperative or intraoperative CT imaging study. Utilizing navigation systems, surgeons can get real-time 3D anatomy of the spine structure and proximity of neurovascular structures in the surgery field. The endoscopic electromagnetic navigation system consists of a field generator, a patient tracker and registration tool, a sensor wire, a processing computer, and compatible TESSYS-ISEE instruments.[7] From our early experience, we conclude that intraoperative navigation for full-endoscopic spine surgery assists with the determination of an optimal skin entry point and, the correct angle of the approach trajectory. This is in particular important in anatomically constrained areas such as lower cervical spine or transforaminal approaches to the L5/S1 foramen. Moreover, it provides real-time information regarding location and orientation of the surgical field throughout the procedure.

4.3 Indications for Intraoperative Navigation

Intraoperative navigation can replace the intraoperative use of fluoroscopic imaging in all full-endoscopic procedures. It greatly facilitates posterior endoscopic approaches in the lower cervical spine where the shoulders typically obscure the spine on lateral fluoroscopy and make determination of the correct spine level cumbersome. It is in particular useful to optimize skin entry point and trajectory for L5/S1 transforaminal approaches in patients with high iliac crests. Intraoperative navigation also facilitates execution of full-endoscopic procedures in the setting of severe degenerative changes, scoliosis, and revision surgeries that obscure anatomical landmarks. In these cases, continuous real-time information regarding the location and orientation of the endoscope assists with safe progression of the procedure obviating the need for frequent AP and lateral fluoroscopic imaging.

4.4 Preoperative Planning and Positioning

Before the surgical procedure, CT scans with a slice thickness of 1 mm are obtained from the surgical area and a 3D reconstruction is made. The CT dataset is stored in DICOM (digital imaging and communications in medicine) format for the 2D/CT alignment and registration process in the navigation system. The intraoperative C-arm should be compatible with electromagnetic navigation and calibrated at regular intervals according to the manufacturer's recommendations. The patient is placed in the prone position on a special, nonmetallic, carbon fiber OR (operating room) table to prevent interference. The field generator is placed gluteal or ventral to the patient, thereby allowing the electromagnetic field to encompass the entire surgical field (▶ Fig. 4.4 **a**). Two K-wires are anchored to the spinal column by driving them approximately 2 cm deep into the bone of the caudal index-level spinous process or into the iliac crest. The

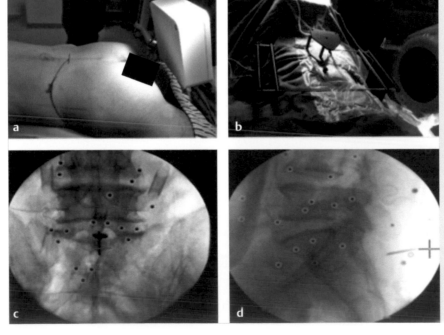

Fig. 4.4 **(a)** The electromagnetic field generator is placed at the gluteal side of the patient. The patient tracker is attached to the spinous process. **(b)** For patient registration, the mapper bridge is placed just next to the localizer. At least 17 markers of the mapper bridge are identified on **(c)** anteroposterior and **(d)** lateral fluoroscopic images.

patient tracker/registration tool is attached to the K-wires at a 5- to 10-mm distance to the skin and the K-wire directly above the localizer cut to avoid interference with subsequent surgical activities. The patient tracker/registration tool firmly attached to the spinal column serves as the reference for the navigation unit in the coordination system (▶ Fig. 4.4 **b**). The mapper bridge that is placed just next to the localizer should be identified on least 17 markers in AP and lateral fluoroscopic images to allow for the most accurate patient registration (▶ Fig. 4.4 **c, d**). The mapper bridge needs to be positioned on the back so that all mapper symbols are green. After lateral and AP images have been taken, any movement of the mapper bridge should be avoided. Then the fluoroscopy images are transferred to navigation using USB (universal serial bus). Once imaging data are loaded, the system automatically performs the registration. The system can correct static errors that are attributable to the position and alignment of the navigation instrument. After confirmation of the registration, the intraoperative 2D images are used to match the preoperative CT data. Then navigation is carried out virtually, in real time, within the 3D dataset. In the navigation mode, the sensor wire (joimax, Intracs) can be mounted into different instruments such as an 18-G needle, guiding rod, tubular retractor, red disposable reamer, and endoscope.

4.5 Surgical Technique

The entire surgery may be performed under local anesthesia or optional narcotic sedation. The stylet is removed from the 18-G needle, and the sensor wire is inserted into the needle with Luer connection locked. The needle is registered by placing it onto the patient tracker/registration tool (▶ Fig. 4.5 **a**). A total

amount of 15 to 30 mL of 0.5% lidocaine is infiltrated in the puncture trajectory through the needle (▶ Fig. 4.5 **b**). Real-time navigation with inline views or target views is used to aim for the target area. Thus, an optimal approach corridor can in many cases even be accomplished for narrow L5/S1 foramina with a high iliac crest (▶ Fig. 4.5 **c,d**). A puncture guidance angle is provided during needle targeting, and green is displayed when the angle is correct. Then the surgical procedure is performed as follows:

1. A guide wire is passed through the 18-G needle, and the needle is removed.
2. A small skin incision is made at the entry point of the guide wire using a no. 11 blade.
3. The guiding rod is registered by placing it onto the registration tool.
4. The guiding rod is inserted over the guidewire with the inline views toward the superior articular process.
5. A half-serrated working tube is introduced over the guiding rod, which is withdrawn once the superior articular process is palpated with the working tube.
6. A reamer with a handle is attached to the half-serrated working cannula (▶ Fig. 4.6 **a**).
7. A sensor wire is inserted into the irrigation channel of the endoscope. Following registration of the endoscope, it is inserted (▶ Fig. 4.6 **b**).
8. Ventral osteophytes of the superior articular process can be resected safely under the inline navigation views and removed by forceps under endoscope image shown on the navigation views (▶ Fig. 4.6 **c,d**).
9. After the foraminoplasty, forceps are used to resect the ipsilateral ligamentum flavum (▶ Fig. 4.7 **a,b**).
10. The half-serrated working tube is exchanged for a standard transforaminal working cannula.

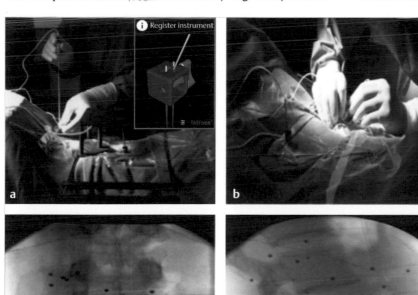

Fig. 4.5 (a) The 18-G needle is placed onto the patient tracker/registration tool until the needle symbol is shown in the top right corner (inset depicts a screenshot during the registration process). (b) For the procedure, a total amount of 15 to 30 mL of 0.5% lidocaine is injected along the approach trajectory. Real-time inline navigation provides guidance to aim for the target area on (c) anteroposterior and (d) lateral views.

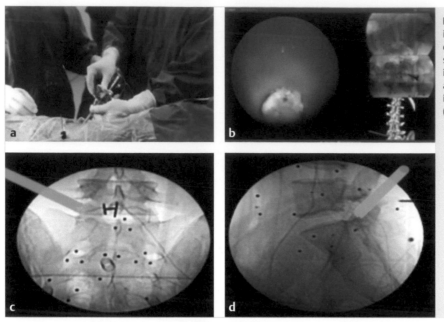

Fig. 4.6 **(a)** A bone reamer with handle is introduced into the half-serrated working cannula. **(b)** The endoscope is registered using a sensor wire placed onto the irrigation canal and inserted into the working cannula. The superior articular process can be resected safely under the inline navigation **(c)** anteroposterior and **(d)** lateral views.

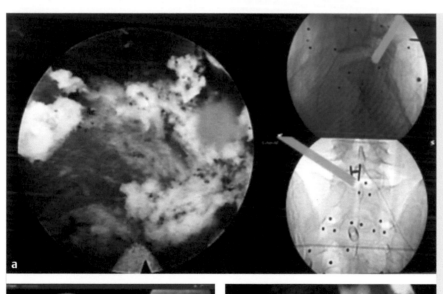

Fig. 4.7 After the foraminoplasty, the ventral surface of the partially resected superior articular process is seen. **(a)** Intraoperative navigation depicts the location of the endoscope. **(b)** The ipsilateral ligamentum flavum is removed using a curette. **(c)** The diskectomy is performed until the nerve root is adequately decompressed.

11. Following the exchange of the working tube, the location of the endoscope is confirmed with the navigation.
12. The diskectomy is performed until the nerve root is adequately decompressed (▶ Fig. 4.7 **b**).

4.6 Conclusion

Intraoperative navigation provides 3D real-time spatial information for access planning and execution of the surgical procedure. Future studies are needed to investigate the impact of navigation on the learning curve and gains in safety by reducing radiation exposure for both patient and surgeon.

4.7 Pearls and Pitfalls

- The skin at the site of the reference array should not be under any tension.
- The reference array needs to be safely secured onto the bone and not touched or bent during the procedure.
- The surface of the target area should always be used to confirm accuracy of the registration. If there is any doubt regarding accuracy, obtain an intraoperative fluoroscopic image for confirmation of accurate registration.

References

[1] Hahn P, Oezdemir S, Komp M, et al. A new electromagnetic navigation system for pedicle screws placement: a human cadaver study at the lumbar spine. PLoS One. 2015; 10(7):e0133708

[2] Hahn P, Oezdemir S, Komp M, et al. Navigation of pedicle screws in the thoracic spine with a new electromagnetic navigation system: a human cadaver study. BioMed Res Int. 2015; 2015:183586

[3] Sagi HC, Manos R, Park SC, Von Jako R, Ordway NR, Connolly PJ. Electromagnetic field-based image-guided spine surgery part two: results of a cadaveric study evaluating thoracic pedicle screw placement. Spine. 2003; 28(17): E351–E354

[4] Kim CW, Lee YP, Taylor W, Oygar A, Kim WK. Use of navigation-assisted fluoroscopy to decrease radiation exposure during minimally invasive spine surgery. Spine J. 2008; 8(4):584–590

[5] Sanai N, Berger MS. Glioma extent of resection and its impact on patient outcome. Neurosurgery. 2008; 62(4):753–764, discussion 264–266

[6] Mezger U, Jendrewski C, Bartels M. Navigation in surgery. Langenbecks Arch Surg. 2013; 398(4):501–514

[7] Xiong C, Li T, Kang H, Hu H, Han J, Xu F. Early outcomes of 270-degree spinal canal decompression by using TESSYS-ISEE technique in patients with lumbar spinal stenosis combined with disk herniation. Eur Spine J. 2019; 28(1):78–86

5 Endoscopic Instruments

Saqib Hasan and Christoph P. Hofstetter

5.1 Introduction

Endoscopic surgery originated in the early 19th century with the invention of rudimentary cystoscopes. Within the next century, endoscopic technology spread to many surgical subspecialties. While arthroscopic surgery gained widespread adoption by the late 20th century, full-endoscopic spine surgery has only recently garnered increasing popularity. This is primarily due to recent advances in illumination, high-definition imaging, adjunctive technologies, and novel endoscopic tools. The proposed benefits of endoscopic surgery include similar outcomes compared to traditional spine surgery while reducing invasiveness, complication rates, and cost. Potential disadvantages of endoscopic surgery include increased operating times, a steep learning curve, and the need for new equipment. The decision to utilize endoscopy must involve consideration of the potential benefits of this method weighed against its limitations.

5.2 Working-Channel Endoscope

The working-channel endoscope contains an optical system and conduit for illumination, which are sealed within the rigid tube. There are two basic optical designs: a rod-lens system or coherent optical fiber bundles (▶ Fig. 5.1). The gross majority of spinal working-channel endoscopes use a rod-lens system as it allows for superior optical resolution (PANOVIEW/VERTEBRIS Stenosis, Wolf; Tessys/ilessys, joimax; Spine TIP, Storz). Optical fibers allow for tighter packaging and are used in the smallest spinal working-channel endoscopes utilized, for example, in anterior cervical procedures (CESSYS, joimax). Fiberoptic images have the disadvantage that the images have a pixelated appearance since each individual "pixel" constitutes an individual fiber. Regardless of the design, the endoscope carries light from a source into the body cavity and the subsequent light reflected from the illuminated anatomy is transmitted back to the endoscope and directed into a video camera.

Endoscopes utilized for full-endoscopic spine surgery contain a working channel within the endoscope shaft, which allows passage of specialized endoscopic tools to the operative field (▶ Fig. 5.1). This is in contrast to "endoscope-assisted" surgeries such as endoscopic transsphenoidal surgery or arthroscopic surgery where the instruments are not passed through the endoscope but instead through separate access routes. For transsphenoidal surgeries, tools are passed via the contralateral nares and for arthroscopic surgeries tools are passed through a port inserted via a separate skin incision. Utilization of endoscope-assisted technique is possible in the spine and is referred to as biportal endoscopic spine surgery.

Full-endoscopic spine surgery requires the creation of an artificial working space to allow for visualization of spinal pathology. This is in contrast to transsphenoidal surgery, which utilizes the nasal cavity/sphenoid sinus or arthroscopic surgery, which uses joint cavities as working space. In full-endoscopic spine surgery, creation of an artificial working space is aided by the serial dilators, tubular retractor, continuous irrigation, and surgical tools. First, serial dilators generate an approach corridor through the soft tissue, which is secured by the tubular retractor. The soft tissue between the tip of the tubular retractor and the spinal pathology is resected with grasping forceps and with the bipolar cautery ("tucking soft tissue away under the edges of the tubular retractor"; for technique, see Chapter 9). The artificial working space is maintained by the bevel of the tubular retractor, which avoids soft-tissue creep, and by the continuous fluid irrigation. Anatomical structures within that space are illuminated and directly visualized with high definition. Hence, the spinal endoscope has four primary components: optical system, illumination, irrigation channels, and working channel.

5.2.1 Optical System

- Endoscopes are differentiated on the basis of optical characteristics, which include the lens diameter, field of view, and angle of inclination (▶ Table 5.1).

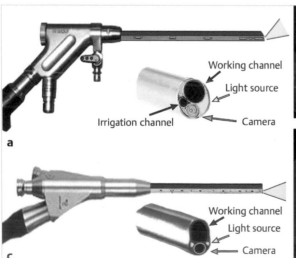

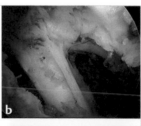

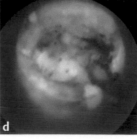

Fig. 5.1 Examples of different optical systems used for working-channel endoscopes. (a) A rod-lens (*green*) working-channel (*red*) endoscope with a 25-degree angle of view. (b) A rod-lens optical system allows for high-resolution images. (c) A fiberoptic system allows for extremely compact design resulting in an extremely small outer diameter of the working-channel endoscope. This endoscope provides a straight-on view. (d) Images obtained with a fiberoptic system have a pixelated appearance since each individual "pixel" constitutes an individual fiber.

In figure (a): Working channel, Light source, Irrigation channel, Camera

In figure (c): Working channel, Light source, Camera

Table 5.1 Various working-channel endoscopes and specifics

	Manufacturer	Endoscope designation	Length (mm)	Outer diameter (mm)	Working-channel diameter (mm)	Irrigation channel diameter (mm)	Angle of view (degrees)	Tubular retractor inner/outer diameter (mm)	
Anterior cervical diskectomy	joimax	CESSYS	100 and 150	3.9	2.1	None	0	4.0/4.8	Fiberoptic endoscope (40,000 pixels)
	Wolf	Cervical diskoscope	150	?	3	1.5 × 1	25	Need working tube ID/OD	
Posterior cervical diskectomy	joimax	CESSYS Dorsal	68	7.3	4.7	1.5 × 2	15	7.5/8.5	Any interlaminar endoscope can also be used for this application
Transforaminal endoscopic thoracic diskectomy	joimax	TESSYS Thx	120	5.8	3.1	1.4 × 2	45	5.9/6.9	
Transforaminal endoscopic lumbar diskectomy	joimax	TESSYS	171	6.3	3.7	1.5 × 2	30	6.5/7.5	
	Wolf	PANOVIEW Plus (transforaminal)	205	5.9	3.1	1.85 × 1	25	6.0/7.0	
	Storz	Spine TIP (transforaminal)	255	6.6	3.6	1.6 × 2	25	6.8/7.8	
Trans-SAP	joimax	TESSYS Pro	171	7.3	4.7	1.5 × 2	30	7.5/8.5	
	Wolf	PANOVIEW Plus (transforaminal)	207	6.9	4.1	1.85 × 1	25	7.0/8.0	
	Storz	Spine TIP (posterolateral)	180	6.1	2.9	1.6 × 2	15	6.2/6.9	
Interlaminar endoscopic lumbar diskectomy	joimax	iLESSYS Pro	150	7.3	4.7	1.5 × 2	15	7.5/8.5	
	Wolf	PANOVIEW Plus (interlaminar)	165	6.9	5.6	1.5 × 1	25	7.0/8.0	Uses space between round tubular retractors and elliptical endoscope as egress port
	Storz	Spine TIP (interlaminar)	180	6.6	3.6	1.6 × 2	25	7.2/7.9	
LE-ULBD	joimax	iLESSYS Delta	125	10.0	6.0	2.0 × 2	15	10.2/13.7	
	Wolf	VERTEBRIS Stenosis	177	9.3	5.6	1.85 × 2	20	9.5/10.5	

Abbreviation: ID, interior diameter; LE-ULBD, lumbar endoscopic unilateral laminotomy for bilateral decompression; OD, outside diameter.

- The diameter of the lens determines the size of the endoscope as well as the field of view. The lens diameter determines the outer diameter of the endoscope together with the size of the working channel. The field of view can vary from 1.7 to 7 mm.
- The angle of inclination is defined as the angle between the long axis of the endoscope and a line perpendicular to the lens. The angle of view can vary from 0 to 45 degrees for spinal working channel endoscopes.
- The selection of the proper endoscope depends on the type of approach, segment of the spine, as well as the type of pathology being addressed (▶ Table 5.1). The are several special endoscopic features pertinent for various approaches:
  - Anterior cervical approaches require a small outer endoscope diameter (4 mm) to reach the pathology via the collapsed disk space.
  - Transforaminal endoscopic thoracic diskectomy is facilitated by a larger angle of view (45 degrees) since the ribcage does not allow for a shallower approach angle.
  - Transforaminal endoscopic lumbar diskectomy requires a small outer diameter to safely enter the foramen and a 25- to 30-degree angle of view to allow for visualization of exiting and traversing nerve roots.
  - Interlaminar endoscopic lumbar diskectomy allows for a straight-on view of the pathology and requires less angulation of the view compared to the transforaminal route (15–25 degrees).
  - Lumbar endoscopic unilateral laminotomy for bilateral decompression is facilitated by a larger working channel (6 mm), which allows for more efficient resection of degenerative pathology.

5.2.2 Illumination

- A light source port is typically found at the base of the endoscope (▶ Fig. 5.2). A fiberoptic cable from a light source compatible with this port is necessary.
- The light is transmitted via glass fibers to the tip of the endoscope.

5.2.3 Irrigation Channels

- Inflow and egress irrigation channels in the endoscope shaft allow for fluid to constantly circulate through the working area (▶ Fig. 5.2). The ports for inflow and egress irrigation channels are typically located at the lateral aspect of the base of the endoscope. Tubing connects to the inflow port and delivers saline irrigation from a fluid pump. The egress port allows fluid to escape freely. In case of bleeding, the egress port may be temporarily closed.

5.2.4 Working Channel

- The working channel is the tube through which instruments pass (▶ Fig. 5.2). Working-channel sizes range from 2.1 to 6.0 mm depending on the type of endoscope. The working channel limits the size of instruments being used. It determines the outer diameter of the endoscope together with the size of the lens diameter. The ratio of the working channel to the lens diameter and associated outer diameter distinguishes various endoscopic designs (▶ Table 5.2).

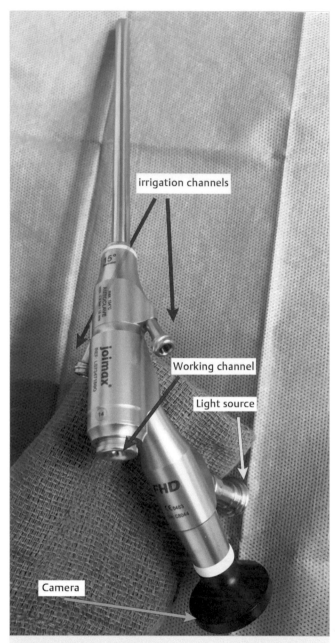

irrigation channels

Working channel

Light source

Camera

Fig. 5.2 Endoscope connections.

- The working-channel lengths of spinal endoscopes can vary from 68 to 255 mm. Working-channel length differs depending on the type of approach. The longest endoscopes are utilized for transforaminal approaches as they have to transgress the flank tissue during the approach. In large morbidly obese patients, the endoscope shaft length of some transforaminal systems might be insufficient to reach the target area. Extra-long endoscopes (Spine TIP [transforaminal], 255-mm length; TESSYS HD Foraminoscope XT, 208-mm length; PANOVIEW Plus [transforaminal] 205-mm length) are available for such cases.
- Endoscopic surgical tools are optimized for the diameter and length of various working-channel endoscopes. They have to be long enough to be advanced beyond the endoscope into

Table 5.2 Various endoscope designs

Endoscope designs				
Brand names	CESSYS	Spine TIP Yess	iLESSYS TESSYS VERTEBRIS Stenosis	PANOVIEW Plus
Characteristics	• Small-diameter fiberoptic endoscope • No irrigation channel	Two irrigation channels	Two irrigation channels	• One irrigation channel • Elliptical design—gap between round tubular retractor and elliptic endoscope serves as egress port

Note: *blue*, irrigation channel; *green*, optics; *red*, working channel.

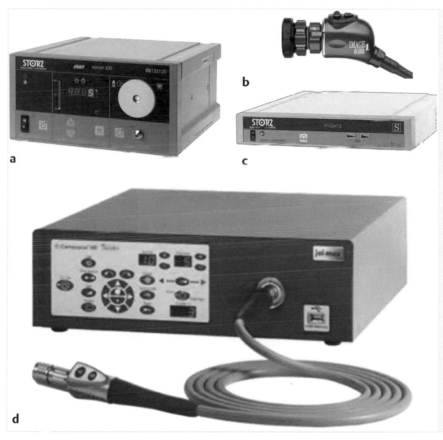

Fig. 5.3 Endoscopic light sources and video systems. **(a)** Endoscopic light source with 300 W (Cold light Fountain XENON 300 SCB, KARL-STORZ). **(b)** Full HD camera head (IMAG1 S Camera Head, KARL-STORZ). **(c)** Digital image processing module (IMAGE1 S CONNECT, KARL-STORZ). **(d)** Combined camera and light source and camera head with intergraded light cable (Camsource HD Twister, joimax).

the surgical field as well as to allow for 360 degrees of rotation to optimize workflow.

5.3 Illumination

The endoscopic working field is typically illuminated by a xenon light source (100–300 W) that is housed on an endoscopic tower (▶ Fig. 5.3 **a**). Fiberoptic cables consisting of bundled glass fibers are utilized to transmit light from the light source to the endoscope. The intensity and quality of light are reduced by the cable length or fiber damage. Fiber breakage is a

routinely observed wear-and-tear issue of light cables. They should therefore be tested at regular intervals.

5.4 Video Equipment

The image obtained via the optical system of the endoscope is recorded by a camera attached to the base of the endoscope (▶ Fig. 5.3 **b**). The image from the camera is digitized into a video signal by a video processor (▶ Fig. 5.3 **c**). The processor accentuates contrast, optimizes colors, and projects the life-image onto a video monitor. The video processor box is typically housed on the endoscopy tower. The video monitor can be directly connected to the cart or it may be integrated into the operating room on mobile supports. With advancements in video processing technology and improved camera resolution, current endoscopic spine systems offer high-definition visualization of spinal anatomy. To reduce the number of boxes on the endoscopic tower and the number of cables that cross into the sterile field, illumination and video equipment may be combined in one unit (▶ Fig. 5.3 **d**).

5.5 Fluid Pump

An essential component of full-endoscopic spine surgery is continuous irrigation. A physiologic solution such as normal saline should be used for irrigation. Continuous fluid irrigation improves visualization of structures, allows for removal of debris, and also provides gentle retraction of neural elements. Only fluid pumps designed for full-endoscopic spine surgery can be used as they allow for precise control of the flow rate and hydrostatic pressure within the working area (▶ Fig. 5.4 **a**). Typically, specialized tubing is required, which allows for pumping of the fluid as well as monitoring of flow and pressure (▶ Fig. 5.4 **b**). Our initial default settings are 50 mmHg of pressure at a rate of 0.4 L/min. In order to facilitate clearance of debride or to improve visualization in cases of diffuse bleeding, the irrigation pressure and the flow rate may be increased. As a general rule, the irrigation pressure should be lower than the patient's diastolic blood pressure. Optimal irrigation management is a key component to perform successful endoscopic surgery as it plays a role in the management of bleeding, visualization, and debris clearance.

5.6 Surgical Instruments

The surgical instruments utilized in full-endoscopic spine surgery are analogous in function to those utilized for minimally invasive or traditional spine surgery. The key distinguishing features of instruments designed for working-channel endoscopic spine surgery are their diameter and length. Endoscopic surgical instruments must be narrow enough to fit through a specific diameter working channel. Moreover, endoscopic instruments must be longer than the lengths of the working channel in order to allow us to reach pathology in the surgical field. Additionally, the handle should be designed to allow for utilization of the instruments at any rotational angle in relation to the endoscope. In order to increase the width of the surgical field, some endoscopic instruments may have flexible tips. Conceptually, endoscopic surgical instruments can be divided into categories based on the specific task that needs to be completed.

5.6.1 Instruments for Targeting and Creating an Approach Corridor

Fluoroscopic localization and targeting during endoscopic spine surgery are very similar to minimally invasive tubular spine surgery. Fluoroscopic imaging is utilized to localize the index spinal level and the target area to plan the entry point and appropriate approach trajectory. Instruments such as a long spinal needle, Jamshidi needle, or trocar are used to dock on the approach-specific target area utilizing fluoroscopic guidance (▶ Fig. 5.5 **a**). Once the target area is reached, the tip of the instrument provides valuable tactile feedback that allows for characterization of the consistency (bone vs. disk) as well as the surface characteristics (shape and orientation) of the target area. This information is helpful for making fine adjustments to the docking location as well as for a seamless endoscopic exposure of the target area. A guidewire is then used as a place holder at the docking site and sequential dilators are used to

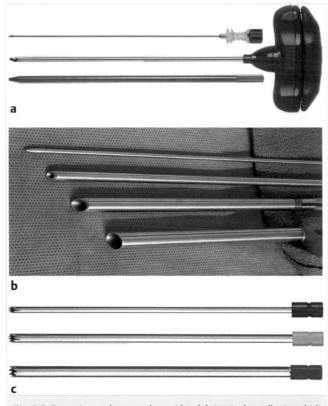

Fig. 5.5 Targeting and approach corridor. (**a**) A spinal needle, Jamshidi needle, or trocar may be used for docking. (**b**) Serial dilators are used to create a working corridor through soft-tissue planes. (**c**) Bone reamers may be used to perform a foraminoplasty.

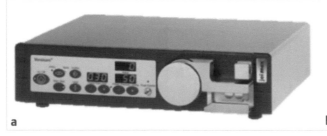

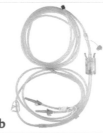

Fig. 5.4 Fluid irrigation system. (**a**) An example of a spine pump: joimax Versicon Spine Pump provides fluid flow with a pressure set at 0 to 100 mm Hg at 0 to 750 mL/min. (**b**) Specialized tubing allows for monitoring of pressure and flow.

create a larger working corridor via soft-tissue planes (▶ Fig. 5.5 **b**). For transforaminal procedures, trephines, bone reamers, or osteotomes may be used to remove bone along the surgical corridor (▶ Fig. 5.5 **c**).

5.6.2 Instruments to Maintain the Artificial Working Space

Once the approach corridor has been created, a tubular retractor is brought in (▶ Fig. 5.6). The tubular retractor has several functions: First, it helps create an artificial working space to allow for visualization of spinal pathology. Soft-tissue creep is minimized by an optimized bevel seal with the surface of bony structures. A more acutely angulated bevel is utilized for lumbar interlaminar approaches compared to cervical approaches reflecting the different lamina slope and width angles between these spinal segments (see Chapter 7). Interlaminar tubular retractors that remain outside the spinal canal have typically a straight angulated bevel design (▶ Fig. 5.6 **a**). This design optimizes retraction of paraspinal muscles and soft tissue. Tubular retractors designed for interlaminar approaches, which are advanced into the spinal canal, have a slightly curved bevel design (▶ Fig. 5.6 **b**). The curved bevel design avoids impingement of the nerve root during rotational retraction. Moreover, it enhances protection of the retracted neural elements as the tip of the bevel has a wider area compared to a straight angulated bevel design. Tubular retractors designed for the transforaminal approach have a much more angulated bevel in order to minimize the mass effect onto the exiting nerve root. Moreover, soft-tissue creep is less of an issue within the confinements of the intervertebral foramina (▶ Fig. 5.6 **c**). Certain tubular retractors designed for application in severely stenotic foramina have a very slim bevel and serve mainly as anchorage for the operative corridor (▶ Fig. 5.6 **d**).

5.6.3 Instruments for Dissection and Removing Tissue

Given that the diameter of the working channel is limited, surgical instruments must be highly efficient and allow for reach of off the axis structures.

5.6.4 Radiofrequency Instruments

- Radiofrequency instruments can be used for cutting and shrinking soft tissues and for developing surgical planes. They also play a vital role in obtaining hemostasis (▶ Fig. 5.7).
- Radiofrequency instruments generate a high-frequency electromagnetic current at their tip, causing heat to be generated by the resistance to current passage through tissue. These instruments can be monopolar or bipolar and the tip may be flexible to allow multiple access angles.
- Monopolar systems allow current flow from the tip of the instrument to a grounding pad on the patient, using the path of least resistance, and generate heat at the tissue closest to the tip. Bipolar devices permit passage of current between two electrodes at the tip of the instrument, heating the tissue between them.
- The specific effect of the instrument is dependent on the amount of heat transferred. Low level of heat cause denaturation of collagen fibers and shrinking of tissues, while higher levels destroy collagen and can be used for tissue ablation and debridement. Low levels of heat are typically utilized for coagulation of blood vessels.

5.6.5 Lasers

- The use of lasers is controversial in full-endoscopic spine surgery. A laser is a tool for tissue ablation and its use is not a prerequisite for performing endoscopic spine surgery.

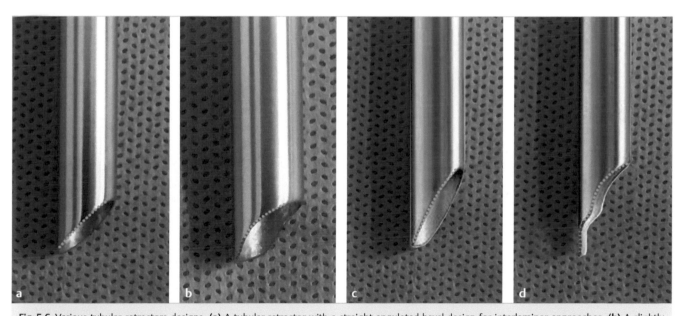

Fig. 5.6 Various tubular retractors designs. **(a)** A tubular retractor with a straight angulated bevel design for interlaminar approaches. **(b)** A slightly curved bevel design for work within the spinal canal is depicted. Note that the area of the bevel contacting the nerve during retraction has a steeper angle in order to avoid impingement of the nerve. **(c)** A tubular retractor with a straight acutely angulated bevel for transforaminal approaches. **(d)** Tubular retractor for the treatment of severely stenotic foramina with a slim tip (*red dotted line*) as anchorage point.

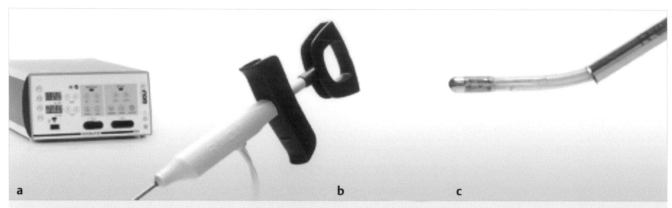

Fig. 5.7 Radiofrequency instruments. **(a)** A 4-MHz radiofrequency device (Surgi-Max PLUS RF, Wolf). **(b)** Hand piece of the radiofrequency probe. **(c)** Articulatable bipolar electrode for coagulation and ablation.

Conceptually, a laser is a beam of monochromatic light with a specific energy level. The amount of energy, area of focus, wavelength, pattern of pulsation, and type of laser determine the effect of the laser on the tissue. One advantage of the laser over radiofrequency instruments is the ability to quickly and thoroughly ablate soft tissues.

- The types of lasers available for use in full-endoscopic spine surgery include holmium:yttrium aluminum garnet (Ho: YAG), erbium:yttrium aluminum garnet (Er:YAH), neodymium:yttrium aluminum garnet (Nd:YAG), and potassium titanyl phosphate (KTP) lasers. All of these lasers can be transmitted through flexible optic fibers, unlike the CO_2 laser, which is used in other surgical subspecialties. Ho: YAG lasers are the most commonly used lasers in endoscopic spine surgery and is often used in the form of a side-firing laser with rotational capabilities. Many surgeons primarily utilize lasers for superficial soft-tissue dissection and work within the annulus. The differences between using one laser over another is based on surgeon preference.
- While lasers may expedite workflow with efficient soft-tissue ablation, their use must be weighed against potential risk of iatrogenic neurologic injury, aseptic diskitis, and laser-induced osteonecrosis. Moreover, powerful side-firing lasers can easily damage the optical system of working-channel endoscopes, and the acquisition and maintenance costs of lasers are significant.

5.6.6 Motorized Instruments

Shaver

A motorized shaver consists of a pair of cylinders, one inside the other with a matching window. The window of the inner cylinder has sharp edges that can cut tissue as it spins within the outer cylinder. Suction is attached to the outer cylinder, which draws tissue into the inner cylinder for tissue resection. Shavers range in diameter, angles, and type of blades. Control of the motorized shaver can be accomplished via manual hand control of the shaft or via a foot pedal.

Burr

A motorized burr that is analogous to the burrs used in open spine surgery is utilized (▶ Fig. 5.8 **a**). Burrs vary by the type of material used (tungsten carbide or diamond), the diameter of the burr, and the angulation and flexibility of the tip (▶ Fig. 5.8 **b**). Larger diameter burrs allow for more efficient bone resection as progression of the burr is not impeded by the drill shaft. Diamond burrs are highly efficient in full-endoscopic spine surgery as they are continuously rinsed and cooled in full-endoscopic spine surgery. Diamond drills also minimize bony bleeding. Articulating burrs provide access to more-difficult-to-reach off-axis targets and are particularly useful for transforaminal surgery.

5.6.7 Basic Surgical Instruments

There are endoscopic iterations of almost all instruments found in traditional spine surgery. Instruments such as elevators, sharp dissectors, nerve hooks, and curettes can be used to dissect tissue planes and mobilize neural structures. Micropunches and Kerrison rongeurs are utilized to resect tissue. Pituitary rongeurs, grasping forceps, and cup forceps are used to retrieve soft tissue (▶ Fig. 5.9).

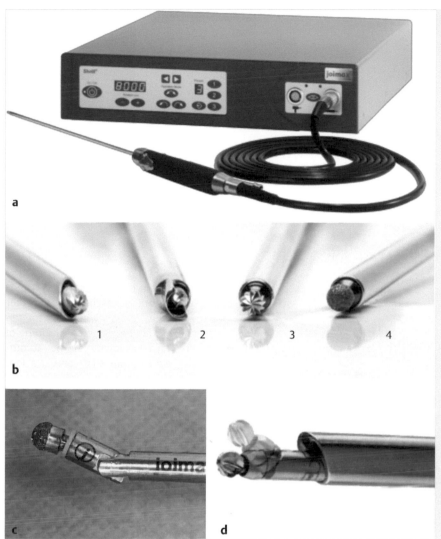

Fig. 5.8 Powered burrs. **(a)** Example of a drill unit (Shrill, joimax). **(b)** Examples of various burrs: (1) oval burr with lateral soft-tissue hood, (2) oval burr with lateral and frontal soft-tissue hood, (3) round cutting burr, and (4) diamond round burr. **(c)** Articulating diamond burr and **(d)** round cutting burr.

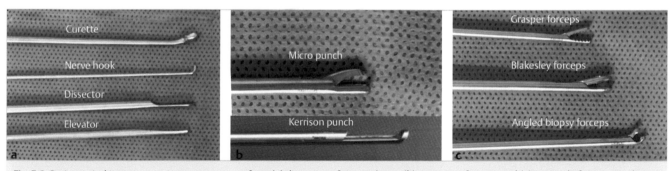

Fig. 5.9 Basic surgical instruments. Instruments to perform **(a)** dissection of tissue planes, **(b)** resection of tissue, and **(c)** retrieval of tissue are shown.

6 Operating Room Setup: The Basics

Saqib Hasan and Christoph P. Hofstetter

6.1 Introduction

Full-endoscopic spine surgery is performed in a standard surgical suite in a hospital or ambulatory surgical center. The operating room must be large enough to accommodate the required endoscopic tower, monitors, and fluoroscopic equipment and should be staffed by operating room personnel trained in full-endoscopic surgery. The basic spinal endoscopic system includes an endoscope, fiberoptic light cable and light source, camera, saline irrigation tubing and pump, video processing unit, video monitors, and C-arm. The endoscope tower should house the light source box, the video processor box, the fluid pump, the radiofrequency box, as well as power for any motorized instruments.

6.2 Operating Room Layout

The layout of the operating suite is very similar to minimally invasive spine surgery (▶ Fig. 6.1). The surgeon typically stands on the side of the affected pathology. The scrub nurse and instrument table are positioned at the base of the patient next to the surgeon. The endoscope tower is located at the base of the patient. The C-arm is positioned opposite the surgeon. Monitors are also opposite to the surgeon and should be at eye level of the surgeon.

6.3 Positioning

The patient can be positioned prone or lateral, depending on the procedure being performed. The lateral position is preferred for awake transforaminal endoscopic lumbar approaches as this position facilitates airway control. Moreover, it allows for performing a straight leg raise test at the end of the procedure. For cases performed under general anesthesia, the prone position is typically preferred as it is a similar setup to minimally invasive

spine surgery. A radiolucent table with a Wilson frame to kyphose the lumbar spine is used to provide larger interlaminar or foraminal working areas. For cervical procedures, the patient's head may be secured with a Mayfield head holder. Secure fixation of the patient's head is imperative for cervical endoscopic unilateral laminotomies for bilateral decompression where any patient motion could lead to injury of the spinal cord. Body warmers are used to maintain appropriate core temperature. This is in particular important given that the continuous irrigation can significantly affect the patient's temperature.

6.4 Equipment Setup

Prior to the procedure, the endoscope should be connected to the light source, camera, and irrigation tubing. Two 3-L 0.9% sodium chloride solution bags are set up in a piggyback configuration connected with a y-connector. This setup allows seamless exchange of empty bags without interrupting the workflow or introduction of air bubbles into the tubing (▶ Fig. 6.2). At the time of setup, all tubing should be flushed with irrigation fluid and clear of air bubbles. The irrigation pressure needs to be adjusted to the height of the operative field, since the selected pressure on the pump produces a particular hydrostatic pressure above the level of the pump. This is in particular important for obese patients who have a higher venous pressure and are elevated higher. Failing to level the irrigation pressure in these patients can be frustrating given that the combination of lower irrigation pressure and increased venous pressure leads to cumbersome venous bleeding. For a quick estimation of the

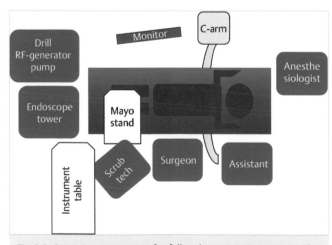

Fig. 6.1 Operating room setup for full-endoscopic spine surgery. The scrub tech is next to the surgeon. The C-arm should be opposite of the surgeon.

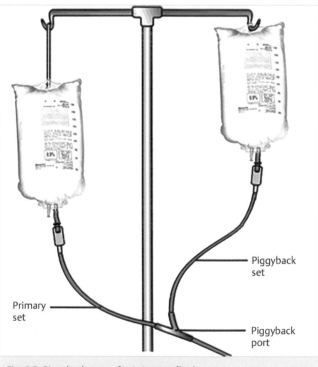

Fig. 6.2 Piggyback setup for irrigation fluid.

available irrigation pressure at the operative field, elevate the endoscope until the irrigation ceases: elevation height in cm × 0.74 = pressure in mm Hg. A suction is utilized to collect egress irrigation fluid from the operative field. The endoscope picture displayed on the monitor is inspected for any problems with picture quality. The white balance function should be performed with a sterile sponge to normalize any color distortion. Motorized instruments should be tested to confirm they are functioning properly prior to use in the patient.

6.5 Operative Field

Capture of egressing irrigation fluid is the main challenge for the operative field in full-endoscopic spine surgery. There are several strategies to prevent fluid puddles on the floor (▶ Fig. 6.3):

- The Ioban drape should produce a tight seal on the skin surrounding the incision site. Applying the drape onto a thoroughly dried skin enhances adhesion. Moreover, skin adhesives can be applied onto the skin before placing the drape to further enhance the seal.
- A pouch should be used wide enough to capture egressing irrigation fluid dripping off the endoscope. A suction is placed into the pouch to continuously retrieve fluid.
- If irrigation fluid leaks from the operative field, floor suction devices may be utilized.

6.6 Staff

Staff should be familiar with the endoscopy cart and be able to perform functions such as adjusting fluid pressure, light source wattage, and record multimedia, and also be able to change radiofrequency and motorized control settings.

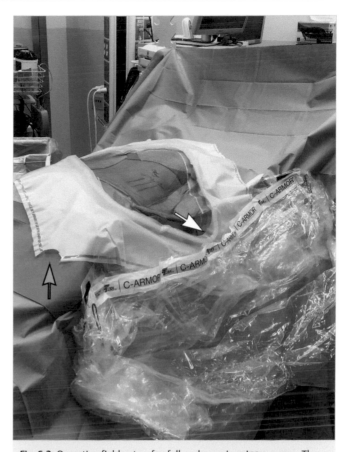

Fig. 6.3 Operative field setup for full-endoscopic spine surgery. The pouch of the drape is wide enough to capture dripping egress irrigation from the endoscope (*white arrow*). A small opening in the pouch is produced as a conduit for the light cable, camera cable, and irrigation tubing.

7 Applied Anatomy for Full-Endoscopic Spine Surgery

Daniel Carr and Christoph P. Hofstetter

7.1 Cervical Spine Applied Anatomy

7.1.1 Posterior Fascia

Posterior approaches to the cervical spine require passage through the paraspinal soft tissue using palpation and fluoroscopy for guidance only. Blunt dissection and dilation through the tissue can be challenging given the multiple muscle layers and fascial planes. The most superficial investing fascia divides around the trapezius muscle, while the prevertebral layer of fascia encircles the deeper muscles of the neck (▶ Fig. 7.1). Rather than transgressing these layers bluntly with downward force and the risk of plunging into the spinal canal, they may be cut sharply with a no. 11 blade (for surgical technique, see Chapters 21 and 22).

7.1.2 Lamina and Ligamentum Flavum

During posterior endoscopic cervical approaches, the posterior bony spinal elements are first encountered with the tip of the trocar. Precise knowledge of the bony surface morphology is essential to safely identify the correct target area using only palpation and fluoroscopic guidance. During advancement of the trocar, serial dilators, and working tube, the juxtaposed edges of index-level laminae serve as the *target area*. The distance between laminae varies greatly depending on individual anatomy, amount of disk collapse, and degree of flexion of the neck and needs to be studied on preoperative imaging studies. Great care must be taken to avoid inadvertent entry into the spinal canal during the initial palpation and dilatation. The anatomy of the laminae varies among individuals and between genders. On average, the lamina of C4 has the lowest height (10.4 mm).[1] The lamina height then gradually increases toward the caudal cervical spine with C7 having an average height of 15.1 mm (▶ Fig. 7.2 **a**). The slope angle of the lamina in

reference to the horizontal plane increases from C3 to C7[1] (▶ Fig. 7.2 **b**). In terms of mediolateral extent, the cervical laminae span from the spinous process medially to the facet laminar line laterally. The width angle at which the two paired laminae meet is approximately 100 degrees from C2 to C7 except at C3, where is its typically larger (▶ Fig. 7.2 **c**).[1] The slope and width angles of the lamina are of importance since they should be roughly matched by the angulation of the bevel of the tubular retractor. This optimizes the seal and minimizes soft-tissue creep.

The cervical ligamentum flavum is a paired structure that meets in the midline and blends with the interspinous ligament.[2] Frequently, there is a sagittally oriented midline cleft, where bilateral ligamenta flava are not entirely fused. The ligamentum attaches at the ventral inferior half of the cranial lamina and the ventral superior edge of the caudal lamina (▶ Fig. 7.3 **a,b**). It spans laterally to the superior articular process (SAP), but typically does not extend into the neural foramen beyond the medial aspect of the pedicle. Laterally, the yellow ligament fuses with the facet capsule and ligaments at the cranial medial edge of the SAP. The cervical yellow ligament is on average 2.2-mm thick and is thinnest at C2–C3.[2] For posterior endoscopic foraminotomies, docking with the working tube is carried out in the lateral aspect of the juxtaposed edges of the index-level laminae. There the laminae transition into the articular processes and form a "**V**"-shaped structure that can be easily visually identified and serves as the target area for this approach (▶ Fig. 7.4).

7.1.3 Facet Joints and Intervertebral Foramen

Facet joints localized from C2 to C7 are diarthrodial synovial joints surrounded by fibrous joint capsules. The articulating surfaces are formed by the inferior articular process of the rostral segment and the SAP of the caudal segment. The joints are

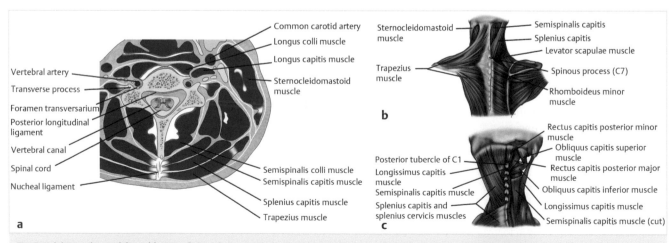

Fig. 7.1 **(a)** Muscles and fascial layers of the of the cervical spine depicted on an axial section. Posterior views of **(b)** superficial and **(c)** deep neck muscles are shown.

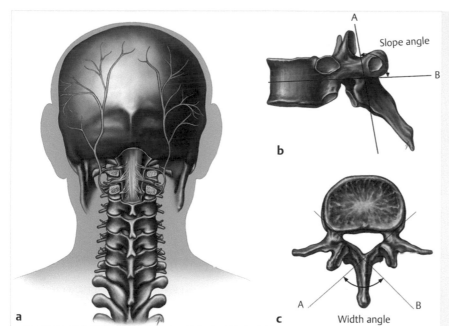

Fig. 7.2 **(a)** Posterior view of the cervical spinal column. Illustration depicting **(b)** the slope angle and **(c)** the width angle of the of the lamina.

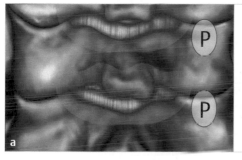
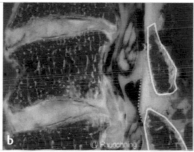

Fig. 7.3 Yellow ligament of the cervical spine. **(a)** Anteroposterior projection of the yellow ligament onto the laminae of the cervical spine. Note that the yellow ligament extends to the mid-portion of the rostral laminae and is attached to the superior edge of the caudal-level lamina (P, pedicle). **(b)** A paramedian sagittal section of the cervical spine reveals the lamina (*white line*) insertion of the yellow ligament (*green dotted line*). (Adapted from Rahmani et al 2017.[2])

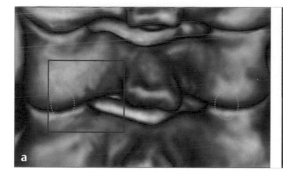
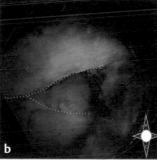

Fig. 7.4 First visualized bony landmark for a posterior endoscopic cervical foraminotomy. **(a)** Illustration depicting the location of the caudal pedicle in relation to the posterior superficial bony anatomy (*red box* depicted in panel b). **(b)** Adjacent edges of the index laminae transition into the articular processes forming a "V"-shaped structure (*green dotted line*).

inclined at an angle of 45 degrees from the horizontal plane and 85 degrees from the sagittal plane.[3] The intervertebral foramen is confined by the uncus in front, the facet joint (SAP) behind, and pedicle below.[3] The medial and lateral borders of the foramen are confine by the mediolateral extent of the inferior pedicle. On X-rays, the center of the caudal pedicle can be estimated in general as 2 mm inferior to the facet joint line and 5 mm medial to the facet joint line.[4] The pedicle angulation is 70 to 80 degrees from the lateral mass. The facet width for the subaxial cervical spine of both inferior and superior articulating processes is 11 to 13 mm on average. The caudal pedicle of each foramen has a constant reliable relationship to the exiting spinal nerve. The exiting nerve root is found directly along the rostral aspect of the caudal pedicle.[5] The transition of caudal lamina to pedicle can therefore serve as a reliable bony landmark to identify the exiting nerve root during a posterior foraminotomy. Moreover, the nerve root is adequately decompressed once the posterior endoscopic cervical foraminotomy reaches the lateral aspect of the caudal pedicle. The caudal index-level pedicle serves therefore as the *principal anatomical landmark* for this procedure.

Cervical spinal nerves are composed of dorsal and ventral roots, which join lateral to the foramen near the vertebral artery (▶ Fig. 7.5). In the cervical spine, the spinal nerve roots exit directly above the inferior pedicle of each foramen with no measurable distance in cadaveric studies. The same is true in regard

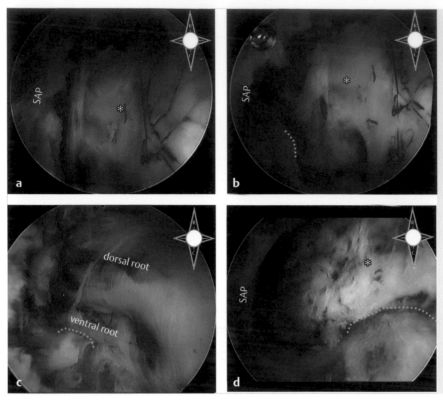

Fig. 7.5 Intraoperative view during a posterior cervical foraminotomy. **(a)** Proximal area of the exiting nerve root (*asterisk*) is exposed. **(b)** Upon further resection of the medial aspect of the superior articular process (SAP), the outline of caudal lamia–pedicle transition becomes visible (caudal pedicle, *green dotted line*). **(c)** Cervical nerve roots consist of a ventral and a dorsal root. **(d)** The exiting nerve root (*asterisk*) is found directly adjacent to the superior aspect of the caudal index-level pedicle.

to the thecal sac medially where there is also no space between the medial pedicle and dura.[5] The ventral root is closer to the pedicle inferiorly and the uncinate process anteriorly. The dorsal root follows a more posterior and superior tract closer to the SAP and terminates at the dorsal root ganglia that is found extra-foraminally and just lateral to the vertebral artery.[6]

7.2 Thoracic Spine Applied Anatomy

7.2.1 Lamina and Ligamentum Flavum

During thoracic endoscopic unilateral laminotomies for bilateral decompressions, the posterior bony spinal elements are first encountered with the tip of the trocar. The thoracic laminae are greater in both height and thickness compared to the other segments of the spine. The thoracic laminae become greater in height in the lower thoracic spine, with T11 being the tallest (25.1 mm). The lamina of T2 is the thickest with an average thickness of 5 mm.[1] The ligamentum flavum attaches at the ventral inferior half of the cranial lamina and the ventral superior edge of the caudal lamina. The ligamentum flavum height and width increase gradually from the upper and lower thoracic spine. Moreover, the ventral lamina height covered by ligamentum flavum increases from upper (T1–T2: 31.7%) to the lower levels (T12–L1: 41.7%).[7]

7.2.2 Facet Joints and Intervertebral Foramen

Thoracic intervertebral foramina are similar in configuration to lumbar foramina except for a smaller size and incorporation of

the rib. At T2–T9, the rib head is adjacent to the disk space and extend beyond the disk space superiorly. At T10, the rib head is at the level of the disk space and at T11 and T12, the rib head is more inferior and does not overlap with the entire disk space[8] (▶ Fig. 7.6). Thoracic spinal nerves are centered in the foramen, located 2 to 3 mm below the superior pedicle and 2 to 3 mm above the inferior pedicle of the foramen.[9]

Thoracic pedicles are composed of a shell of cortical bone, which is thicker medially than laterally, and a core of cancellous core. The cancellous core takes up to 79% of the entire dimension of the pedicle.[10] Thoracic pedicles are taller than they are wide. The facet joints in the thoracic spine are oriented in the coronal plane. For transforaminal endoscopic thoracic approaches, the SAP of the caudal index-level serves as the *target area*. The average width of the SAP from lateral to medial is 10 to 12 mm except at T1, which is about 15 mm.[9] The caudal index-level pedicle is considered the *principal anatomic landmark* for the transforaminal endoscopic thoracic approach as it allows for reliable and safe identification of the spinal cord.

7.3 Lumbar Spine Applied Anatomy

7.3.1 Lamina and Ligamentum Flavum

During interlaminar endoscopic lumbar approaches, the posterior bony spinal elements are first encountered with the tip of the trocar. While the facet joint can undergo significant hypertrophic changes, the inferomedial margin of rostral index-level lamina constitutes a reliable *target area*. The lumbar laminae measure 20.4 to 22.7 mm in height, except for the L5 lamina, which is significantly shorter (16.6 mm).[1] Thus, at L5/S1, a

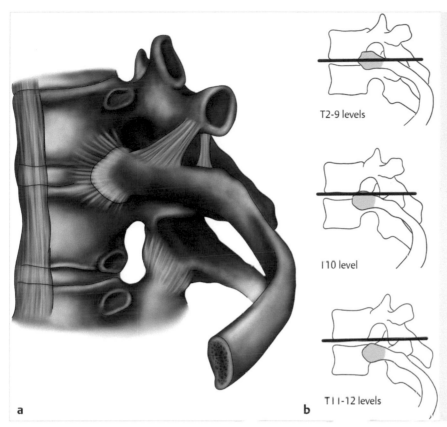

T2-9 levels

I10 level

T11-12 levels

a

b

Fig. 7.6 Relationship of the rip head to the intervertebral thoracic foramina. **(a)** Lateral depiction of the thoracic spine revealing the relationship of the rib with the foramen. Note the radiate ligament and the superior costotransverse ligament anchoring the rib to the vertebral body. **(b)** The position of the rib head in relation to the intervertebral foramina differs in the upper thoracic spine (rib head covers part of the intervertebral disk) compared to the lower thoracic spine (rib head is below the level of the disk).

larger interlaminar window is only covered by yellow ligament and initial docking of the tubular retractor may be carried out on the yellow ligament. The lamina width increases progressively from 11.5 mm at L1 to 15.7 mm L5.[1] This has important implications on the choice of endoscope. Lamina width of 15 mm or more allows for the efficient use of a central stenosis-type endoscopes (endoscope diameter of 10 mm). The lamina thickness is greatest in the upper lumbar levels, which may make bony decompression more time-consuming. The slope angle of lumbar laminae in reference to the horizontal is approximately 115 degrees except for L3, which has a slope angle of plane of 140.1 degrees in males.[1] Given the steep L3 slope angle, initial docking with the trocar on inferomedial lamina edge can be challenging, as it may be difficult to palpate the narrow inferomedial edge with the tip of the trocar. Moreover, the trocar can easily slip off onto the dorsal surface of the lamina following docking. Thus, steady bone contract needs to be maintained from the beginning of docking with the trocar, dilation, placement of tubular retractor to visualization of the inferomedial lamina edge with the endoscope. The width angle of the inferior lamina is 93.2 degree at L1 and increases to 119.1 at L5. The slope and width angles are important parameters as they determine the seal between the dorsal surface of the lamina and the bevel of the tubular retractor. A good seal minimizes tissue creep. Moreover, the width angle also determines the trajectory for the contralateral laminotomy. Given that the angle is more acute in the upper lumbar spine in combination with more narrow interpedicular distance, the need for undercutting the spinous process and contralateral angulation of the endoscope necessary to reach the contralateral lateral recess is much less in the upper lumbar compare to the lower lumbar spine.[11,12]

The lumbar yellow ligament constitutes a ligamentous arch, which spans the interlaminar space (▶ Fig. 7.7 **a**). The yellow ligament consists of a superficial and a deep layer, which are firmly adherent to each other. The superficial portion is light yellow in color and approximately 2.5- to 3.5-mm thick and blends into the interspinal ligament. This is of importance during the interlaminar approach since the interspinal ligament can easily be mistaken for the yellow ligament. This can be avoided by paying close attention to the endoscope trajectory and careful visualization of the yellow ligament attachment along the lamina. The superficial portion of the yellow ligament attaches to the base of the spinous process and the inferomedial edge of the rostral lamina and spans to the superior edge and the posterosuperior surface of the caudal lamina (▶ Fig. 7.7 **b,c**). The superficial layer of the yellow ligament can be safely removed after the laminotomy along the inferior edge of the rostral lamina and the medial aspect of the inferior articular processes are completed. Resection is carried out with a large Kerrison rongeur in a rostrocaudal direction until the superior edge of the caudal lamina is reached. At that point, the deep portion of the yellow ligament, which is slightly darker in color and approximately 1-mm thick, is exposed. The deep portion of the yellow ligament spans from the ventral surface of the rostral lamina to the anterosuperior surface of the caudal lamina and anteromedial surface of the SAP.[13] At L1–L2, the rostral extend of the ligamentum is approximately 50% of the rostral index level lamina height, whereas it is almost 70% at L3–L5. Likewise, the inferior extent of the deep L1/L2 ligamentum is 1 to 2 mm below the rostral edge of L2 and at L5–S1 approximately 5 to 6 mm beyond the superior edge of S1.[14] The ligamentum also extends further laterally following the tip of the

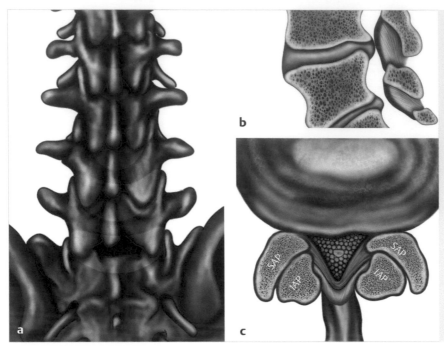

Fig. 7.7 Yellow ligament of the lumbar spine. **(a)** Reconstructed 3D CT image with an overlay of the yellow ligament (*yellow*). **(b)** Illustration of the lumbar yellow ligament on a sagittal section. The deep portion of the yellow ligament is slightly darker in color. Axial section of the lumbar spine depicts attachment of the yellow ligament on the medial aspect of the facet joint. The deep portion is attached to the anteromedial portion of the superior articular process (SAP). **(c)** The superficial portion is attached to the medial aspect of the inferior articular process (IAP).

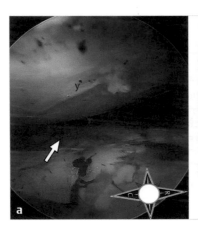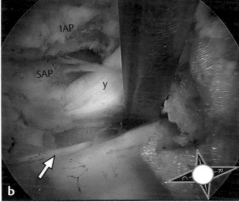

Fig. 7.8 (a) Intraoperative view of a stenotic contralateral L4/L5 lateral recess. Note the traversing L5 nerve root (*arrow*) within the lateral recess that is confined posteriorly by the yellow ligament (y) covering the anterior portion of the facet joint. **(b)** Partial removal of the yellow ligament (y) reveals the L4/L5 facet joint formed by the inferior articular process (IAP) and the superior articular process (SAP). The traversing nerve root is marked with an *arrow*.

SAP and fusing with the facet capsule more laterally. The medial border of the pedicle to the lateral border of the ligamentum flavum increases from 6.5 mm at L1–L2 to 11 mm at L5–S1.[14] The lamina attachment of the yellow ligament serves as the *principal anatomical landmark* for interlaminar endoscopic lumbar decompression surgery as it guides bony decompression.

7.3.2 Lateral Recess

The lateral recess constitutes the entrance zone for lumbar nerve roots entering the nerve root canal. The lateral recess is localized underneath the SAP and is confined by anterior and posterior walls. The anterior wall is formed by the annulus of the disk and the posterior wall by the SAP covered by ligamentum flavum[15] (▶ Fig. 7.8). The anteroposterior measurements for the lateral recess gradually decreases from L1 (9.1 mm) to L4 (6.0 mm). At L5, the anteroposterior lateral recess height is approximately 6.1 mm.[16]

7.3.3 Kambin's Triangle

The foraminal annular window overlying the dorsolateral disk was first described by Kambin.[17] The triangular foraminal annular window is bordered superiorly by the exiting nerve root, inferiorly by the vertebral body endplate of the caudal index-level segment, posteriorly by the ventral surface of the SAP, and medially by the traversing nerve root (▶ Fig. 7.9). The surface of the annulus is covered by adipose tissue. The annulus itself contains sensory nerves and vasculature, necessitating local analgesia and hemostasis if this corridor is chosen into the disk space. An anatomic study revealed that Kambin's triangle is on average 18.9-mm wide and 12.3-mm high.[19] Another anatomical study proposed that the maximum safe diameter of transforaminal tubular retractor was on average 8 mm at the L1–L4 spinal segments, while the diameter was reduced to 7 mm at L4–S1.[20] While these measurements may serve as a rough estimate, the dimensions of the actual safe working zone are

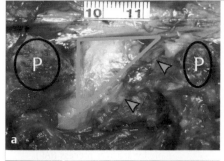
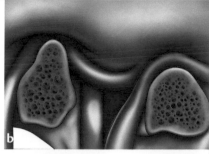
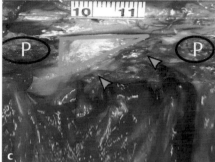
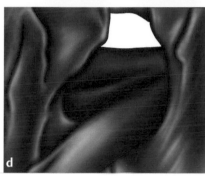

Fig. 7.9 Straight-on posterior view of Kambin's triangle at L4/L5. **(a)** Note that the triangle is delineated by the width of the index-level pedicles between the exiting and traversing nerve roots. **(b)** An illustration of the photograph seen in **(a)**. **(c)** Photograph and **(d)** illustration of a posterolateral view of the working triangle of L4/L5.[18] Note the deceased size of the triangle compared to the straight-on view.

greatly impacted by the approach angle, degree of hypertrophy, and the location of the exiting nerve root within the foramen. ▶ Fig. 7.9 depicts reduction of the size of safe working zone with a more shallow approach angle (more distance of the skin incision to the midline). For these reasons, we recommend Kambin's triangle as a *target area* only under optimal conditions. In these cases, the needle can be inserted into the annulus in the medial portion of the Kambin's triangle, in line with the medial one-third of the pedicle. This is the safest target area with an average distance to the exiting nerve root of approximately 11.9 mm.[18]

However, in most cases we recommend to perform the annulotomy under continuous endoscopic visualization.

7.3.4 Intervertebral Foramen

Lumbar intervertebral foramina are delineated by adjacent vertebral pedicles superiorly and inferiorly, the posteroinferior margin of the superior vertebral body, the posterior intervertebral disk, and the posterosuperior margin of the inferior vertebral body as the anterior limit, and the ligamentum flavum as well as the SAP as posterior boundaries[21] (▶ Fig. 7.10 **a**). Height estimates of lumbar intervertebral foramina varies greatly in the current literature. Thus, Hasegawa and colleagues determined the lumbar foraminal height to range between 20 and 22 mm.[22] Stephens and colleagues measured the lumbar foraminal height to be 13.6 to 16.6 mm.[21] The size of the spinal nerves in the lumbosacral size increases from L1 to S1 and then decreases from S1 to S5. Nerve root size difference is primarily due to increase in size of the diameter of dorsal and ventral roots as well as an increase in the number of dorsal rootlets from L1 to S1 and subsequent decrease in diameter and quantity from S1 to S5.[16] The nerve roots are located in the superior portion of the intervertebral foramen. The ratio between cross-sectional area of nerve root in relation to cross-sectional area of

the foramen is significantly increased at L5–S1 compared to the rest of the lumbar spine.[22] This ratio is further increased in the cases of foraminal stenosis.[22]

Intraforaminal ligaments and fatty tissue surround the nerve roots and provide support.[23] An array of ligaments suspend the nerve root from the periosteum. As mentioned earlier, the yellow ligament also extends into the foramen along the ventral aspect of the inferior articular process and the SAP[16] (▶ Fig. 7.10). Thus, the superodorsal aspect of the foramen is covered with yellow ligament. The percentage of foramen covered with ligamentum increases from 62.8% at L1–L2 to 76.4% at L5–S1.[14] When disk degeneration occurs, disk bulges into the foramen, the facet joint slides posteriorly causing buckling of the ligamentum and subsequent nerve compression (▶ Fig. 7.10). Importantly, caudal to the attachment of the yellow ligament, the "empty zone" is found. It is a small area in the inferodorsal aspect of the foramen where the ventral bony surface of the SAP forms the posterior border of the foramen. The empty zone constitutes 34% of the dorsal aspect of the foramen at L1/L2 and decreases to 24% at L5/S1. The empty zone serves as a gateway into the lateral recess. The ventrolateral surface of the SAP serves as the *target area* for the trans-SAP approach. The foraminal yellow ligament is a reliable landmark to identify the exiting nerve root that is located just ventral to it.

7.3.5 Pedicle Morphology

Pedicle width and height are generally larger in males than in females. On average, pedicle width increases from 8.1 mm at L1 to 17.2 mm at L5. Pedicle height remains relatively constant at about 14 mm on average for males and about 11 to 12 mm for females throughout the lumbar spine.[24] The caudal index-level pedicle serves as the *principal anatomical landmark* for transforaminal lumbar approaches.

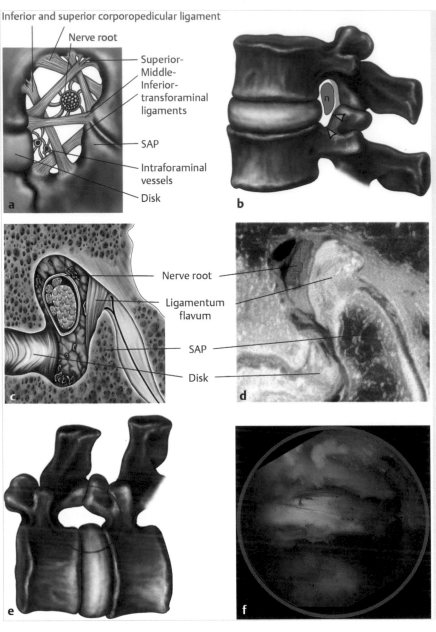

Inferior and superior corporopedicular ligament

Nerve root

Superior-
Middle-
Inferior-
transforaminal
ligaments

SAP

Intraforaminal
vessels

Disk

a

b

Nerve root

Ligamentum
flavum

SAP

Disk

c

d

e

f

Fig. 7.10 Lumbar intervertebral foramina. **(a)** Intraforaminal ligaments provide support for the exiting nerve root. **(b)** The dorsal aspect of the rostral foramen is lined by the *yellow* ligament, while there is a small empty zone at the pedicle—superior articular process (SAP) angle (*green arrowheads*). **(c)** The lumbar spinal nerves are located in the rostral area of the foramen and are surrounded by perineural fat tissue that contains ligaments and blood vessels. **(d)** Degenerative subluxation of the SAP may lead to impingement of the exiting nerve root. **(e)** Transforaminal view of the traversing nerve root. **(f)** The field of view depicted in **(e)** is outlined by a red circle.

References

[1] Xu R, Burgar A, Ebraheim NA, Yeasting RA. The quantitative anatomy of the laminas of the spine. Spine. 1999; 24(2):107–113

[2] Rahmani MS, Terai H, Akhgar J, et al. Anatomical analysis of human ligamentum flavum in the cervical spine: special consideration to the attachments, coverage, and lateral extent. J Orthop Sci. 2017; 22(6):994–1000

[3] Demondion X, Lefebvre G, Fisch O, Vandenbussche L, Cepparo J, Balbi V. Radiographic anatomy of the intervertebral cervical and lumbar foramina (vessels and variants). Diagn Interv Imaging. 2012; 93(9):690–697

[4] Ebraheim NA, Xu R, Knight T, Yeasting RA. Morphometric evaluation of lower cervical pedicle and its projection. Spine. 1997; 22(1):1–6

[5] Xu R, Kang A, Ebraheim NA, Yeasting RA. Anatomic relation between the cervical pedicle and the adjacent neural structures. Spine. 1999; 24(5):451–454

[6] Pech P, Daniels DL, Williams AL, Haughton VM. The cervical neural foramina: correlation of microtomy and CT anatomy. Radiology. 1985; 155(1):143–146

[7] Ahmadi SA, Suzuki A, Terai H, et al. Anatomical analysis of the human ligamentum flavum in the thoracic spine: clinical implications for posterior thoracic spinal surgery. J Orthop Sci. 2018

[8] Moro T, Kikuchi S, Konno S. Necessity of rib head resection for anterior discectomy in the thoracic spine. Spine. 2004; 29(15):1703–1705

[9] Ebraheim NA, Xu R, Ahmad M, Yeasting RA. The quantitative anatomy of the thoracic facet and the posterior projection of its inferior facet. Spine. 1997; 22(16):1811–1817, discussion 1818

[10] Kothe R, O'Holleran JD, Liu W, Panjabi MM. Internal architecture of the thoracic pedicle. An anatomic study. Spine. 1996; 21(3):264–270

[11] Vanharanta H, Korpi J, Heliövaara M, Troup JD. Radiographic measurements of lumbar spinal canal size and their relation to back mobility. Spine. 1985; 10(5):461–466

[12] Hinck VC, Clark WM , Jr, Hopkins CE. Normal interpediculate distances (minimum and maximum) in children and adults. Am J Roentgenol Radium Ther Nucl Med. 1966; 97(1):141–153

[13] Olszewski AD, Yaszemski MJ, White AA , III. The anatomy of the human lumbar ligamentum flavum. New observations and their surgical importance. Spine. 1996; 21(20):2307–2312

[14] Akhgar J, Terai H, Rahmani MS, et al. Anatomical analysis of the relation between human ligamentum flavum and posterior spinal bony prominence. J Orthop Sci. 2017; 22(2):260–265

[15] Lee CK, Rauschning W, Glenn W. Lateral lumbar spinal canal stenosis: classification, pathologic anatomy and surgical decompression. Spine. 1988; 13(3): 313–320

[16] Arslan M, Cömert A, Açar HI, et al. Lumbosacral intrathecal nerve roots: an anatomical study. Acta Neurochir (Wien). 2011; 153(7):1435–1442

[17] Kambin P, Gellman H. Percutaneous lateral discectomy of the lumbar spine: a preliminary report. Clin Orthop Relat Res. 1983; 174:127–132

[18] Hardenbrook M, Lombardo S, Wilson MC, Telfeian AE. The anatomic rationale for transforaminal endoscopic interbody fusion: a cadaveric analysis. Neurosurg Focus. 2016; 40(2):E12

[19] Mirkovic SR, Schwartz DG, Glazier KD. Anatomic considerations in lumbar posterolateral percutaneous procedures. Spine. 1995; 20(18):1965–1971

[20] Wimmer C, Maurer H. Anatomic consideration for lumbar percutaneous interbody fusion. Clin Orthop Relat Res. 2000(379):236–241

[21] Stephens MM, Evans JH, O'Brien JP. Lumbar intervertebral foramens. An in vitro study of their shape in relation to intervertebral disc pathology. Spine. 1991; 16(5):525–529

[22] Hasegawa T, An HS, Haughton VM, Nowicki BH. Lumbar foraminal stenosis: critical heights of the intervertebral discs and foramina. A cryomicrotome study in cadavera. J Bone Joint Surg Am. 1995; 77(1):32–38

[23] Akdemir G. Thoracic and lumbar intraforaminal ligaments. J Neurosurg Spine. 2010; 13(3):351–355

[24] Attar A, Ugur HC, Uz A, Tekdemir I, Egemen N, Genc Y. Lumbar pedicle: surgical anatomic evaluation and relationships. Eur Spine J. 2001; 10(1):10–15

8 Principles of Full-Endoscopic Surgical Technique

Christoph P. Hofstetter

8.1 Progression of Full-Endoscopic Spine Surgery

Traditional surgical approaches typically progress in three steps with quite remarkable consistency among different specialties. First, the general area of pathology is localized with intraoperative imaging, and an appropriate standard surgical approach is performed. During the approach, the surgeon manually palpates the operative field and recognizes tactile features of surgical landmarks and pathology. The obtained three-dimensional perception allows the surgeon to tailor the surgical exposure and to gain direct visualization of the target area.

Progression of full-endoscopic spine surgery follows the same steps. However, given the minimal size of the operative field, a higher level of spatial resolution and precision is necessary to allow for a seamless workflow. Similar to traditional spine surgery, the appropriate spinal segment is localized utilizing intraoperative fluoroscopy. Additionally, full-endoscopic spine surgery requires localization of a radiographically well-defined *target area* with *intraoperative imaging*. Once radiographically visualized, the target area is approached with a needle/trocar allowing for *palpation* of target-specific consistency and surface features. For example, the inferomedial edge of the rostral index-level lamina serves as the target area for the interlaminar endoscopic lumbar approach. The round surface of the lamina and the inferomedial edge can typically be readily appreciated by palpation. For a trans-superior articular process (trans-SAP) approach, the SAP of the caudal index level serves as the *target area*. The ventrolateral orientation of the SAP is palpated and the advance of the needle into the SAP monitored on anteroposterior (AP) and lateral fluoroscopic images. Palpation allows the surgeon to generate a three-dimensional appreciation of the surface features of the target area. This conceived three-dimensional perception is crucial for a seamless transition to *direct visualization* of the target area. Importantly, following soft-tissue dilation with serial dilators, the edge of the lamina (target area) is palpated one more time with the bevel of the tubular retractor. Thus, the surgeon knows exactly where the target area is located in the surgical field. Now the tubular retractor needs to be secured steadily and the endoscope is brought in. Once the endoscope is in place, the bony surface of the target area is exposed and visualized. The precision and accuracy necessary to carry out the progression from imaging to palpation to visualization during full-endoscopic spine surgery is one of the main contributors to the steep learning curve. Several strategies can be applied to facilitate the seamless progression of full-endoscopic spine surgery, which are presented in the following sections.

8.1.1 Radiographic Identification of Target Area

- Obtain well-oriented and undistorted AP and lateral images of the index level.
- Strive for impeccable radiographic depiction of the target area (see Chapter 3).

8.1.2 Transition from Imaging to Palpation

- Careful planning of the incision and trajectory.
- Maintain the angulation of the approach trajectory precisely as planned since a minimal change of trajectory will result in a great deviation of the docking point.

8.1.3 Transition from Palpation to Direct Visualization

- Obtain a three-dimensional appreciation of the surface properties of the target area by palpation with the trocar/needle. This greatly facilitates endoscopic exposure. For example, overgrown facet joints can easily be palpated with the trocar during an interlaminar approach. Once recognized and appreciated, dislodgment of larger-diameter dilators and the working tube can typically be avoided.
- Maintain solid bony contact with dilators and the bevel of the tubular retractor as even a minimal change of the approach trajectory can lead to complete loss of the intended operative field. In this case, the surgeon should restart with the targeting.
- Be proficient in essential surgical tasks, in particular off-axis tissue dissection (see Chapter 9).
- Bone is home—expose bony structures in the surgical field using off-axis tissue dissection.

8.2 Holding the Working-Channel Endoscope

The grip style is different for interlaminar and transforaminal approaches. For interlaminar approaches, the endoscope is held in the web between the index finger and the thumb of the non-dominant hand. Place the tip of the fourth or fifth digits onto the endoscope shaft and maintain the distance between endoscope and tubular retractor (▶ Fig. 8.1 **a**). This controls the depth of the endoscope and distance to target structures. The fourth or fifth digits are also used to rotate the tubular retractor. Alternatively, the depth of the endoscope may be controlled with spacers between working sleeve and the endoscope, which may be helpful for the novice. For transforaminal approaches, the endoscope is held like a pistol, where the index finger is on the working sleeve and the thumb encircles the base of the endoscope from the top along with the third/fourth/fifth digit from the bottom (▶ Fig. 8.1 **b**). The index finger controls the depth of the endoscope and distance to target structures. Moving the endoscope should be a fluid motion in combination with moving the working sleeve. Moving the endoscope without the working sleeve can expose the endoscope to significant mechanical stress, which initially causes blurry areas at the periphery of the

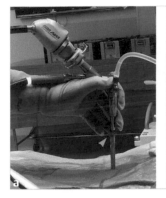
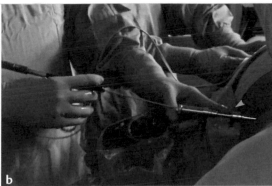

Fig. 8.1 Holding the working-channel endoscope. (a) For interlaminar approaches, the endoscope is held between the index finger and the thumb. The tip of the fourth finger (*green arrowhead*) is placed onto the endoscope shaft to control depth of the endoscope. (b) For transforaminal approaches, the endoscope is held like a pistol. The tip of the index finger (*green arrowhead*) controls the depth of the endoscope.

viewing screen and possible damage to the lens system. In order to avoid damage to the endoscope, it is critical to move the endoscope and tubular retractor in concert.

8.3 Utilizing the Tubular Retractor

Following serial dilation of the soft tissue, the tubular retractor is introduced. Tubular retractors have various designs (see Chapter 5) and serve several functions:

- Maintaining an artificial working space.
- Retracting soft tissue—during in-line and off-axis dissection (see Chapter 9).
- Dissecting soft tissue off the bony surface.
- Mobilize and retract neural elements.
- Elevate scar tissue.

The tubular retractor has a fixed handle. For interlaminar approaches, it points toward the open bevel. For transforaminal approaches, it points away from the open bevel. The handle is operated with the fourth and fifth digit of the nondominant hand and utilized to control rotation and depth of the tubular retractor in relation to the endoscope.

8.4 Continuous Irrigation

The pressure of the continuous irrigation is initially set at approximately 50 mm Hg. In case of venous oozing or large amounts of debride, the pressure can be increased. However, we typically do not increase the pressure beyond the diastolic arterial pressure. Continuous irrigation also facilitates the utilization of diamond burrs as it provides cooling and clearance of debride. The use of bipolar radiofrequency coagulation is also facilitated, since the irrigation fluid acts as a heat sink, thereby mitigating local temperature changes near neural structures. Cold irrigation is generally used to help with hemostasis. In order to avoid hypothermia of the patient, warming devices such as forced air need to be utilized during the operation.

8.5 Working with Tools via the Working Channel

Instruments should be held with the dominant hand. Continuous visualization of the tip of the instruments is facilitated by maintaining instruments and camera at an angle of approxi-

mately 90 degrees. Direct visualization of the instruments can help avoid incidental durotomies or damage to the neural structures. In–out movements need to be carefully controlled, in particular when working around the cervical and thoracic spinal cord. In these cases, we recommend introducing tools while the working channel is pointing at bone. Lateral off-axis instrument movements are facilitated by translation/angulation of the tubular retractor and the endoscope in concert. Lateral forces on instrument shafts should be avoided since they can easily be bent. The goal is a constant coordinated two-handed movement of instruments and the endoscope/tubular retractor.

8.6 Hemostasis

Bleeding is best controlled by prevention. Hemostasis should be meticulous throughout the procedure and the surgical field should be kept clean. Unattended small bleeders add up, diminish visibility, and greatly hamper identification and visualization of a major bleeder should it occur. Whenever possible, tissue should be coagulated with the radiofrequency probe prior to resection with the Kerrison rongeur or micro-punches to minimize bleeding. Diamond burrs help minimize bone bleeding during bony decompression. The irrigation pressure should be leveled for the height of the operative field. For more extensive endoscopic procedures such as unilateral laminotomy for bilateral decompressions (ULBDs), the irrigation fluid can be supplemented with epinephrine (one vial of epinephrine [1 mg] per 3-L bag of irrigation fluid [normal saline]).

8.6.1 Areas of Frequent Bleeding

- Dorsal to the mid part of the lamina:
  - Interlaminar lumbar approach—typically occurs with a deviation of the approach trajectory while attempting to identify the inferomedial lamina edge.
- Small arterial bone bleeders adjacent to facet joints:
  - ULBD in cases with severe joint degeneration.
- Epidural bleeders under the edge of the laminotomy:
  - ULBD, typically caused by bites with the Kerrison rongeur.
- Epidural bleeders under the edge of the lateral recess:
  - ULBD, typically caused by bites with the Kerrison rongeur during the decompression of the contralateral recess.
  - Interlaminar endoscopic lateral recess decompression.

- Perineural arterioles:
  - Interlaminar contralateral endoscopic lumbar foraminotomy.
  - Transforaminal endoscopic lumbar foraminotomy (TELF).
- Epidural venous plexus ventral to the thecal sac near the midline:
  - TELF, during resection of central disc herniations.
  - Transforaminal endoscopic lumbar discectomy (TELD).
- Facet joint vessels at the lateral aspect of the SAP resection:
  - TELF.
  - TELD.

If bleeding occurs and the bleeding vessel is visible, the bipolar coagulation can be utilized for hemostasis. The bipolar cautery works most efficiently by compressing the bleeding vessel with the tip and activating coagulation at the same time. In case of bone bleeding, the bipolar cautery is sometimes not very effective. Alternatively, the area can be sealed with the diamond burr or compressed with a Kerrison rongeur. If there is vigorous bleeding and visibility is lost, the following steps should be applied:

- Do not move your endoscope (the bleeding is at the location of the last surgical maneuver).
- Manually close the irrigation egress port.
- Add rubber sealer on the end of the tubular retractor and the working channel of the scope to minimize fluid egress.
- Increase irrigation pressure.
- Advance the endoscope toward the bleeding source to facilitate visualization of the bleeder.
- Inject 5,000 units of thrombin with a spinal needle into the working channel—hold pressure for a couple of minutes. Inject FLOSEAL (Baxter) into the working channel.

9 Essential Tasks of Full-Endoscopic Spine Surgery

Christoph P. Hofstetter

9.1 Create a Working Space

In contrast to arthroscopy or laparoscopy, full-endoscopic spine surgery does not have a natural body cavity to work in. The working space is therefore artificial and needs to be created. The tubular retractor serves as a guardian of this working space from surrounding paraspinal muscles and soft tissue. Depending on the type of approach, the bevel design of tubular retractors varies (see Chapter 5). The strategy to create an artificial working space to allow for visualization of spinal pathology is similar for all endoscopic approaches. Once the endoscope is introduced, the soft tissue within the tubular retractor is resected in-line utilizing grasping forceps. Ideally, this maneuver exposes some bony surface of the target area, for example, the ventrolateral aspect of the superior articular process (SAP) during the trans-SAP approach or the inferomedial edge of the rostral lamina during the interlaminar approach. The bone exposure is then widened utilizing off-axis dissection with the bipolar cautery. The bipolar cautery shaft is curved and squeezing the pistol grip moves the tip away from the longitudinal axis of the scope (▶ Fig. 9.1 **a–c**). By squeezing the pistol grip in combination with retracting the instrument shaft, a lateral off-axis motion of the bipolar tip can be achieved. Utilizing the maneuver in conjunction with the tubular retractor, efficient generation of an artificial working space and widening of the exposure can be achieved.

9.2 Defining a Bony Edge

For the interlaminar approach, the inferomedial edge of the lamina that has been palpated with the trocar and bevel of the tubular retractor needs to be visualized. Utilizing a micropunch with the straight jaw slightly advanced into the yellow ligament and the open jaw facing the lamina, muscle tissue and connective tissue are scraped off the lamina edge (▶ Fig. 9.2 **a**). This maneuver is carried out from the base of the spinous process to the inferior aspect of the inferior articular process. The bipolar radiofrequency probe is then used to remove residual soft tissue and to better delineate the edge of the lamina (▶ Fig. 9.2 **b**). Utilizing a diamond burr, bone may be resected along the edge of the lamina (▶ Fig. 9.2 **c**) and thus the yellow ligament and its lamina attachment unambiguously identified (▶ Fig. 9.2 **d**).

9.3 Optimizing Off-Axis Reach

Given the longitudinal working channel that serves as conduit for all tools, off-axis reach is limited in full-endoscopic spine surgery. While articulating tools and burrs facilitate off-axis reach, several key maneuvers can maximize off-axis reach with standard instruments. Several tasks in full-endoscopic spine surgery depend greatly on maximizing off-axis reach:
- Undercutting of the lateral recess during unilateral laminotomy for bilateral decompression.
- Decompression of the foramen during interlaminar contralateral endoscopic lumbar foraminotomy.
- Resection of the ventral SAP during TE-LRD.

To understand optimization of off-axis reach, the surgeon needs to be familiar with the built of the working-channel endoscope and the tubular retractor. If the tubular retractor is advanced past the bony edge, it pushes the endoscope off the bony edge (▶ Fig. 9.3 **a**). Withdrawing the tubular retractor until it rests on the surface of the bony edge allows the endoscope to get closer to the bony edge (▶ Fig. 9.3 **b**). The second maneuver that greatly facilitates off-axis reach is the rotation of the endoscope.

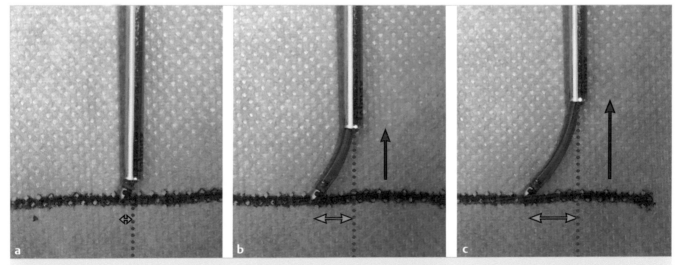

Fig. 9.1 Lateral off-axis utilizing the bipolar cautery. **(a)** In the retracted position, the tip of the bipolar cautery is almost in line with only minimal offset (*green arrow*) from axis of the shaft (*red dotted line*). **(b)** Extending the curved bipolar cautery leads to a lateral movement of the tip. Note that the shaft of the bipolar cautery has been retracted (*blue arrow*). **(c)** Maximum extension of the bipolar cautery further increases the offset (*green arrow*). Note the angulation of the tip of the bipolar also changes.

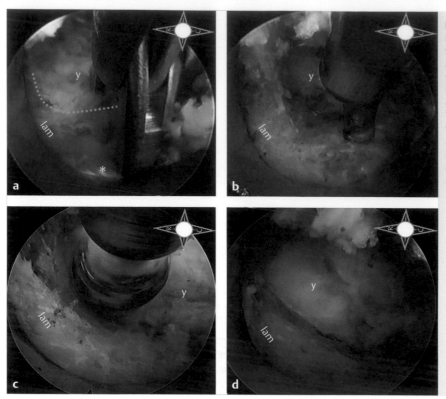

Fig. 9.2 Defining a bony edge. **(a)** During the interlaminar approach, the inferiomedial edge of the lamina (lam; *green dotted line*) is first palpated and then exposed using the micro-punch. The straight jaw is slightly advanced into the yellow ligament (y) and the open jaw is used to scrape off soft tissue from the edge of the lamina (lam). The asterisk indicates the medial aspect of the facet joint. **(b)** Soft tissue along the edge is ablated using the bipolar cautery. Utilizing a diamond burr, **(c)** the lamina is partially resected and **(d)** the yellow ligament and its lamina attachment unambiguously identified.

As discussed in Chapter 5, the location of working channel is excentric in anterior part of the shaft of the endoscope. Thus, rotating the endoscope toward the bony edge minimizes the distance of the working channel toward the edge and greatly facilitates undercutting as well as reaching structures adjacent to the edge (▶ Fig. 9.3 **c,d**). Moreover, this rotational maneuver also facilitates visualization of objects adjacent to the edge as the optics are angled approximately 20 degrees.

9.4 Resection of Soft Tissue In-line with Endoscope

Resection of soft tissue in-line with the endoscope is commonly necessary during full-endoscopic spine surgery. During the interlaminar approach, in-line resection/transgression of the yellow ligament is necessary to enter the epidural space. During the transforaminal approach, resection of the yellow ligament/connective tissue/annulus is necessary to enter the lateral recess and identify the traversing nerve root. The difficulty with this task is that soft connective tissue is resected/transgressed in order to encounter sensitive neural tissue. The most commonly used tool for this task is the micro-punch. Positioning the endoscope in a 90-degree angle in relation to the micro-punch allows continuous visualization of both jaws. Moreover, by gently rotating the instrument with the articulating jaw open, the open jaw functions like a Penfield dissector no. 4 (▶ Fig. 9.4 **a,b**). Thus, the in-line advance of the micro-punch is made utilizing blunt dissection with the open jaw. Closing the instruments typically resects tissue en route. Once a soft tissue layer (such as the yellow ligament) is transgressed with the open jaw, irrigation fluid retracts neural structures (▶ Fig. 9.4 **c**). This maneuver should be utilized with caution if dense

adhesions between soft tissue and neural structures are expected such as in revision surgery, extremely severe stenosis or grade 1 to 2 spondylolisthesis. Resection of soft tissue in line with the endoscope can also be accomplished with other rongeurs such as grasping, cup, or Blakesley forceps; however, the micro-punch allows careful exploration of the border to neural structure and tissue resection without extensive tensile force.

9.5 Off-Axis Resection of Soft Tissue

Resection of soft tissue off-axis is performed using Kerrison rongeurs. This task is very similar to traditional and minimally invasive (MIS) techniques. It is important to coagulate the soft tissue prior to resection in order to avoid cumbersome bleeding. Given the off-axis visualization of the working-channel endoscope, the Kerrison rongeur can be inspected carefully from an approximately 90-degree angle to confirm that the dura is not going to be violated upon taking a bite (▶ Fig. 9.5 **a, b**). An alternative method to resect the yellow ligament during contralateral interlaminar decompression and trans-SAP dorsal lateral recess decompression is the following: the lamina attachment of the yellow ligament is sharply dissected off using the sharp dissection or curette. Detached yellow ligament is then retrieved using grasping forceps.

9.6 Retraction of Neural Elements

During the interlaminar approach, neural elements need to be retracted in order to gain access to the disk space and osteophytes. Prior to retraction, the neural elements need to be

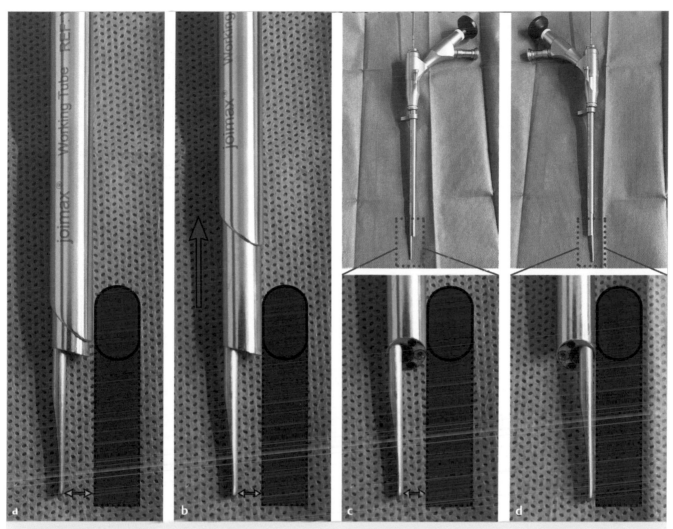

Fig. 9.3 Optimizing off-axis reach. (a) The tubular retractor separates the endoscope from the bony edge (*gray/maroon*) and increases the distance of the tip of the blunt dissector from the lateral wall (*green arrow*). (b) Retracting the tubular retractor brings the shaft of the endoscope into contact with the bony edge and allows the blunt dissector to be closer to the lateral wall (*green arrow*). (c) At this point, the endoscope is directed away from the bony edge and the excentric working channel is at the maximum distance from the bony edge. The lower panel depicts the box indicated with a red dotted line. (d) Turning the endoscope 180 degrees and facing the bony edge brings the working channel into close proximity to the bony edge. In this configuration, the tip of the blunt dissector is adjacent to the lateral wall.

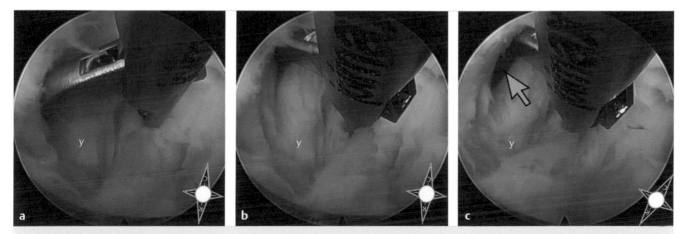

Fig. 9.4 Resection of soft tissue in-line with the endoscope. (a,b) The micro-punch is oriented normal to the fibers of the ligament and advanced with a rotational movement. The articulating jaw of the micro-punch transgresses the yellow ligament (y). (c) Inflowing irrigation fluid enlarges the epidural space (*green arrow*).

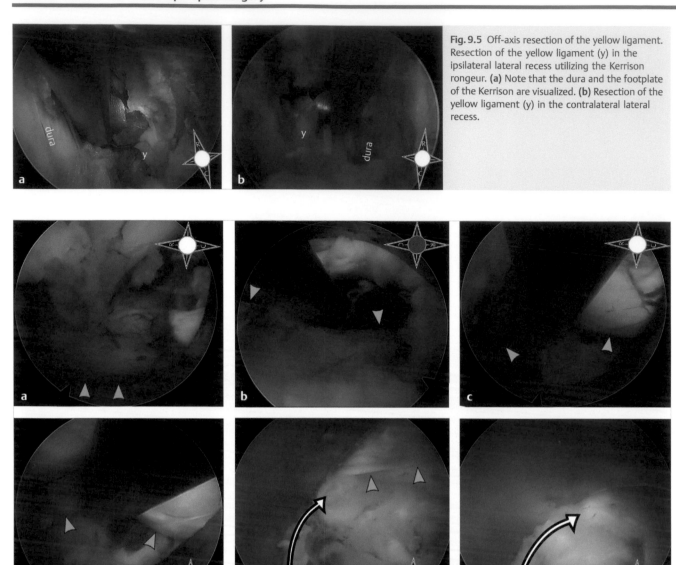

Fig. 9.5 Off-axis resection of the yellow ligament. Resection of the yellow ligament (y) in the ipsilateral lateral recess utilizing the Kerrison rongeur. **(a)** Note that the dura and the footplate of the Kerrison are visualized. **(b)** Resection of the yellow ligament (y) in the contralateral lateral recess.

Fig. 9.6 Retraction of neural elements. **(a)** Nonoptimized view of the lateral margin of the neural elements (*green arrowheads*). **(b)** Optimizing off-axis reach by withdrawing the tubular retractor and rotating the endoscope 180 degrees (note the orientation indicator) leads to a good view of the lateral aspect of the neural elements and allows placing a blunt dissector. **(c)** Rotating the endoscope back 180 degrees, retracting the neural elements with the blunt dissector. **(d)** The tubular retractor is advanced into the spinal canal. **(e)** The tubular retractor is rotated to retract neural elements (*curved arrow*). **(f)** Once the tubular retractor is rotated 180 degrees, the neural elements are completely protected.

mobilized using the blunt dissector. Tethering connective tissue or bridging vessels are coagulated and sharply resected using the micro-punch. Utilizing the optimized off-axis reach technique described earlier, a blunt dissector is utilized to retract the lateral margin of the neural elements (▶ Fig. 9.6 **a–c**). Once the blunt dissector is in place, the endoscope is rotated 180 degrees facing medially. Additional medialization of the neural elements is achieved by tilting the endoscope. Once appropriate retraction has been achieved, the blunt dissector is anchored onto the disk/vertebral body by exerting axial pressure onto the handle. While maintaining pressure onto the blunt dissector,

the endoscope is straightened and the tubular retractor is advanced into the spinal canal with the open bevel facing medially (▶ Fig. 9.6 **d**). While exerting pressure, the tubular retractor is turned 180 degrees to retract neural elements (▶ Fig. 9.6 **e,f**). The direction of rotation is determined by the ease of retraction. If retraction is not easily possible, the following reasons should be considered:

- Residual tethering of neural elements.
- Large extruded disk fragment medial to the neural elements.
- Location of the tubular retractor in the axilla.
- Insufficient undercutting of the medial facet joint.

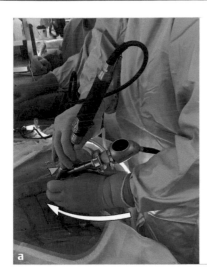
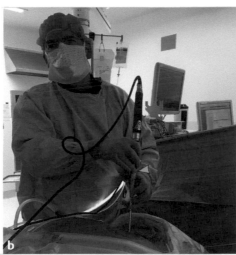

Fig. 9.7 Using the drill. **(a)** Movements of the drill are controlled by angling the tubular retractor in conjunction with the endoscope (*curved white arrow*). The depth of the drill is controlled by placing a fingertip onto the shaft of the drill to prevent nonintentional advance of the instrument (*green arrowhead*; **a,b**). **(b)** Advance of the endoscope is controlled using the same technique (*red arrowhead*).

9.7 Using the Drill

The high-speed drill is invaluable in treatment of degenerative stenotic pathology. Various types of motors and burrs are available (see Chapter 5). For trimming overgrown bone, the burr is used to trim bone in planes rather than engaging the bone at one spot. Engaging the burr at one spot can easily lead to the burr "eating" into the cancellous bone, which causes venous oozing from an area of bone resection that should have not been resected and does not contribute to the bony decompression. As a general rule, bony resection is best carried out along the attachment of the yellow ligament during both interlaminar

and trans-SAP approaches. The burr is moved steadily along the bony attachment of the yellow ligament with minimal pressure onto the bone. Importantly, the movement along the bone is controlled by moving the tubular retractor and the endoscope (▶ Fig. 9.7 **a**). Any torque on the drill handle will bend the drill shaft and will cause heat buildup and eventually failure of the bearings within the drill shaft. The depth of the drill is controlled by the right hand. Nonintentional advancement of the drill should be prevented by placing the tip of a finger onto the drill shaft (▶ Fig. 9.7 **b**). This is imperative during thoracic or cervical decompression surgeries where nonintentional advancement of the drill would cause impingement of the spinal cord.

10 Preoperative Diagnostic Workup

Daniel Carr and Christoph P. Hofstetter

10.1 Introduction

Stringent operative indications are the key to successful surgical outcomes. Given the highly targeted nature of full-endoscopic spine procedures, precise localization of the causative pathology needs to be accomplished utilizing history, static and dynamic imaging, and diagnostic injections. This is in particular important in widespread degenerative spine disease found in the elderly population.

10.2 History and Physical Examination

The history and physical examination serve as the foundation of any diagnostic workup. Determining the exact location and type of radiation of the pain gives important cues regarding the affected spinal segment. Factors that elicit, exacerbate, or alleviate the pain can help determine the type of underlying pathology. Features such as typical dermatomal pattern, pain exacerbation with coughing, sneezing or straining, and pain worse in the leg than the back are all typical findings for nerve root impingement.[1,2] Neurogenic claudication including symptoms such as lower extremity pain, tingling, or cramping when standing or walking is classically reported by patients with central lumbar stenosis. Postural maneuvers that decrease lumbar lordosis such as sitting down or leaning forward (e.g., onto a shopping cart) often alleviate these symptoms as they decrease the in-buckling of the yellow ligament. While not comprehensive, some other features of lumbar spinal stenosis include hypesthesias and paresthesias of the legs and weakness or feelings of heaviness in the legs. Lateral recess syndrome is unilateral or bilateral radiculopathy exacerbated by standing or walking and improved with sitting.[3] There is considerable overlap between lateral recess syndrome and central spinal stenosis and they often occur side by side.

Classic physical examination findings such as positive straight leg raise test are useful in aiding diagnosis but ultimately do not always correlate well with imaging findings.[4] A straight leg raise is considered positive if it occurs between 30 and 70 degrees of hip flexion and suggests L4, L5, or S1 nerve root irritation. Overall, in many surgical series the sensitivity of the straight leg raise test is high and specificity variable; however, in studies utilizing imaging only, there are considerable differences in the sensitivity of straight leg raise test.[4] One author suggested history is the most important component, but dermatomal paresis may aid.[2]

In the cervical spine, Spurling's test has been evaluated in a systematic review and showed a specificity of 89 to 100% and a sensitivity of 38 to 97% in diagnosing cervical radiculopathy. While other findings have not been studied in depth, a positive arm squeeze test, in addition to historical features such as relief with the arm above the head and typical dermatomal findings, may aid in diagnosing cervical radiculopathy.[5] However, it is noted that there appears to be a considerable variation in cervical root dermatomal maps.[6] Symptoms of gait imbalance, bowel or bladder dysfunction, truncal numbness, or sensory level warrant investigation of a spinal cord pathology rather than a nerve root pathology. Red flag symptoms, such as severe recumbent back pain, fever, chills, weight loss, recent trauma, and nighttime pain, should warrant workup for tumor, fracture, or infection.

10.3 Imaging

After the history and physical examination, imaging studies are used to evaluate the soft tissues and bony anatomy of the spine. Magnetic resonance imaging (MRI) is essential to the workup. While MRI occasionally shows only one type of corresponding pathology such as a disk herniation, lateral recess stenosis, or foraminal stenosis, it is exceedingly more common that the spine surgeon is presented with a multilevel degenerative pathological process. It is up to the surgeon to then use the history and physical examination to determine if there are any concordant findings on the imaging.[7]

When evaluating central lumbar stenosis, exact guidelines on measurements for central canal and lateral recess have not been validated. However, obliteration of the cerebrospinal fluid (CSF) space is easily visible to the spine surgeon and absolute stenosis is defined as a canal less than 10 mm in the anteroposterior (AP) diameter. Relative stenosis is when the AP diameter is 10 to 12 mm.[8] The lateral recess is considered stenotic if the AP diameter is less than 2 mm at the medial aspect of the traversing nerve root. One endoscopic surgical series saw a significant difference in the lateral recess between symptomatic and asymptomatic sides by measuring the angle and height. The symptomatic side measured 19.3 degrees, while the contralateral side measured 35.7 degrees. Also, the height was 2.9 mm on the symptomatic side and 5.7 mm on the asymptomatic side.[9]

Many patients have spondylolisthesis in addition to stenosis. In the case of spondylolisthesis, one must determine whether it is a stable or unstable spondylolisthesis. Upright lateral flexion and extension X-rays are utilized to determine if the spondylolisthesis is stable or unstable. The threshold of translational segmental motion to consider it unstable is generally 3 mm.[10] In patients with spondylolisthesis, MRI done in the supine position may underestimate the degree of stenosis, since weight-bearing may cause segmental motion with exacerbation of stenosis. In spondylolisthesis, CT is key to determine whether there are pars defects referred to also as isthmic spondylolisthesis. While there is still considerable debate regarding the role of fusion for stable spondylolisthesis patients,[10] we feel lumbar endoscopic unilateral laminotomy for bilateral decompression (LE-ULBD) is a safe procedure as long as there is no concomitant severe foraminal stenosis.

10.4 Diagnostic Injections

After imaging studies, diagnostic injections are helpful for confirming the segmental origin of radicular extremity pain.

Oftentimes, MRI reveals multilevel pathology or equivocal findings. Sometimes clinical presentation differs from imaging findings, and injections can help differentiate the level of pathology. Selective nerve root blocks (SNRB) performed in the correct way with strict criteria for positive findings can be as accurate as MRI in predicting successful surgical outcomes for lumbar and cervical radiculopathy.[11] It is important to differentiate transforaminal epidural steroid injection as a therapeutic approach for radicular pain from diagnostic injection procedures. SNRB or injections are a diagnostic method, attempting to elucidate if a single nerve root is causing symptoms.[12] The SNRB procedure is variable among providers but generally consists of identification of the nerve root within the foramen utilizing a nerve stimulator or pain provocation, followed by epineural injection of contrast to outline and confirm the nerve root with fluoroscopy, and subsequent use of local anesthetic with patient feedback of pain relief. It has been suggested that the volume of infiltration may affect the selectivity of diagnostic blocks.[12] One prospective controlled trial reports a sensitivity of 57% and specificity of 86% for preoperative SNRB in patients who had complete or near-complete response after one-level surgical decompression.[13]

In conclusion, precise diagnosis of the underlying pathology is essential for successful outcomes with highly targeted full-endoscopic procedures.

References

[1] Verwoerd AJ, Peul WC, Willemsen SP, et al. Diagnostic accuracy of history taking to assess lumbosacral nerve root compression. Spine J. 2014; 14(9):2028–2037

[2] Vroomen PC, de Krom MC, Wilmink JT, Kester AD, Knottnerus JA. Diagnostic value of history and physical examination in patients suspected of lumbosacral nerve root compression. J Neurol Neurosurg Psychiatry. 2002; 72(5):630–634

[3] Ciric I, Mikhael MA, Tarkington JA, Vick NA. The lateral recess syndrome. A variant of spinal stenosis. J Neurosurg. 1980; 53(4):433–443

[4] van der Windt DA, Simons E, Riphagen II, et al. Physical examination for lumbar radiculopathy due to disc herniation in patients with low-back pain. Cochrane Database Syst Rev. 2010(2):CD007431

[5] Thoomes EJ, van Geest S, van der Windt DA, et al. Value of physical tests in diagnosing cervical radiculopathy: a systematic review. Spine J. 2018; 18(1):179–189

[6] Lee MW, McPhee RW, Stringer MD. An evidence-based approach to human dermatomes. Clin Anat. 2008; 21(5):363–373

[7] Saal JS. General principles of diagnostic testing as related to painful lumbar spine disorders: a critical appraisal of current diagnostic techniques. Spine. 2002; 27(22):2538–2545, discussion 2546

[8] Siebert E, Pruss H, Klingebiel R, Failli V, Einhäupl KM, Schwab JM. Lumbar spinal stenosis: syndrome, diagnostics and treatment. Nat Rev Neurol. 2009; 5 (7):392–403

[9] Birjandian Z, Emerson S, Telfeian AE, Hofstetter CP. Interlaminar endoscopic lateral recess decompression-surgical technique and early clinical results. J Spine Surg. 2017; 3(2):123–132

[10] Ghogawala Z, Dziura J, Butler WE, et al. Laminectomy plus fusion versus laminectomy alone for lumbar spondylolisthesis. N Engl J Med. 2016; 374(15): 1424–1434

[11] Sasso RC, Macadaeg K, Nordmann D, Smith M. Selective nerve root injections can predict surgical outcome for lumbar and cervical radiculopathy: comparison to magnetic resonance imaging. J Spinal Disord Tech. 2005; 18(6):471–478

[12] Cohen SP, Hurley RW. The ability of diagnostic spinal injections to predict surgical outcomes. Anesth Analg. 2007; 105(6):1756–1775

[13] Yeom JS, Lee JW, Park KW, et al. Value of diagnostic lumbar selective nerve root block: a prospective controlled study. AJNR Am J Neuroradiol. 2008; 29 (5):1017–1023

11 Interlaminar Endoscopic Lateral Recess Decompression

Christoph P. Hofstetter

11.1 Case Example

A 61-year-old man presents with a 1-year history of right lower extremity radicular pain. The pain radiates from his lower lumbar back, to his right buttock, lateral thigh, and lateral calf. The patient rates the severity as 7 out of 10. On physical examination, the patient has motor weakness of his right extensor hallucis longus (1/5) and foot dorsiflexion (3/5). MRI of the lumbar spine reveals right L4/L5 lateral recess stenosis (▶ Fig. 11.1 **a,b**). The patient underwent a *right L4/L5 interlaminar endoscopic lateral recess decompression*. At the 1-year follow-up, the patient is neurologically intact. The right L5 radiculopathy has resolved. He has minimal persistent numbness of his large toe.

11.2 Indications

The interlaminar endoscopic approach provides access to the ipsilateral recess. This approach utilizes a traditional posterior interlaminar surgical corridor similar to minimally invasive tubular surgery. Thus, the neural elements are encountered first and the risk of injury is minimal. At L5/S1, typically minimal or no bone resection is necessary to gain access to the ipsilateral recess. In lumbar segments above L5/S1, partial removal/undercutting of the lamina and medial aspect facet joint is generally required to gain access to the ipsilateral recess. The need for bone removal is typically less with endoscopic technique compared to minimally invasive surgery since the endoscope provides off-axis panoramic visualization and can therefore look "around corners" rather than requiring a straight line of sight. However, removal of extensive osteophytes and overhanging bone in cases of scoliosis may be time-consuming. Precise planning of the approach angle and meticulous attention to anatomical landmarks help maintain the surgical workflow and minimize the need for bone removal. The interlaminar endoscopic approach is well suited for spinal pathology confined to the bony spinal canal within the medial walls of the pedicles. Subarticular lumbar disk herniations, in particular at L5/S1, are an appropriate indication. Lateral recess stenosis and synovial cysts are additional indications for this approach. The

interlaminar approach constitutes the foundation for the unilateral laminotomy for bilateral decompression and interlaminar contralateral foraminal decompression (see Chapters 14 and 13, respectively). The following pathologies can be treated with either interlaminar or transforaminal approach: subarticular disk herniations, lateral recess stenosis, and certain synovial cysts. The following factors favor the interlaminar approach: lower lumbar segment in particular L5/S1, large interlaminar window, and the need for additional lateral recess or central decompression. For OR setup and patient positioning, see Chapter 6.

11.3 Approach

A thorough review of the preoperative MRI is essential in order to choose the appropriate type of endoscope and approach trajectory. There are two main types of endoscopes for interlaminar approaches: larger endoscope with an outer diameter of approximately 10 mm (iLESSYS Delta, joimax; VERTEBRIS Stenosis, Wolf) or a smaller endoscope with an outer diameter of approximately 7 mm (iLESSYS Pro, joimax; Panoview Plus, Wolf; Spine TIP, Storz; for more technical details, see Chapter 5). The authors suggest the following algorithm to determine the optimal type of endoscope for a particular interlaminar case: If the distance between the spinolaminar angle and the facet joint measured on an axial MRI (▶ Fig. 11.2 **a,b**) is equal or greater than 1.5 cm, the larger endoscope should be considered as it permits more efficient decompression and is less affected by bleeding in the operative field. For patients with a distance of less than 1.5 cm or pathology within the spinal canal such as disk herniations, the smaller interlaminar endoscope is preferred. The second parameter that needs to be determined preoperatively is the optimal rostrocaudal approach angle. An optimal approach angle needs to provide access to spinal canal spanning from the tip of the superior articular process (SAP) to the mid-portion of the caudal index-level pedicle, which constitutes the desired rostrocaudal extent of the lateral recess decompression (▶ Fig. 11.2 **c**). For intraoperative planning of the rostrocaudal approach angle, an anteroposterior (AP) endplate view of the caudal

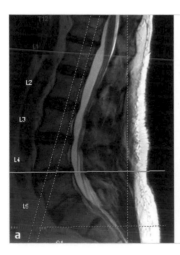
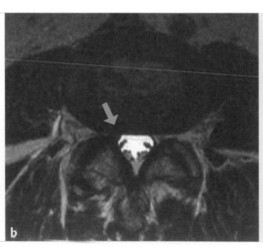

Fig. 11.1 Imaging studies of patient with unilateral L4/L5 lateral recess stenosis. **(a)** Sagittal T2-weighted image of the lumbar spine. **(b)** Impingement of the right L5 traversing nerve root (*green arrow*) is seen in the right lateral recess on a T2-weighted axial image centered on L4/L5 disk.

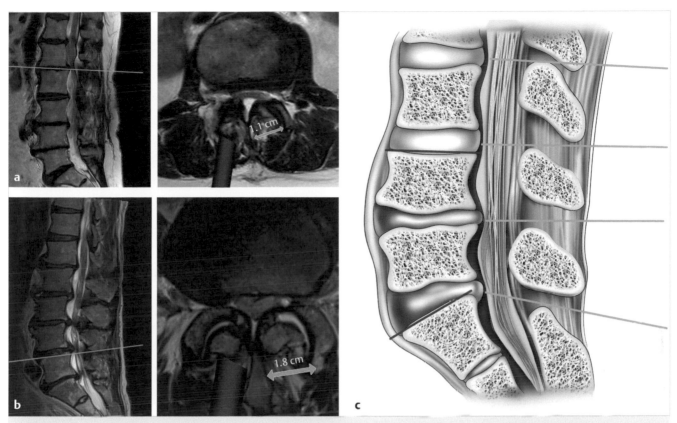

Fig. 11.2 Determination of the appropriate endoscope and rostrocaudal approach angle for various lumbar spinal segments. (a) Axial T2-weighted MR image of the lumbar spine with stenosis at L1/L2. The distance between the spinolaminar angle and the facet joint is 1.1 cm. The *red shape* represents the size of a 7-mm interlaminar endoscope including a tubular retractor. (b) Axial T2-weighted MR image of the lumbar spine with stenosis at L4/L5. The distance between the spinolaminar angle and the facet joint is 1.8 cm. The *red shape* represents the size of a 10-mm interlaminar central stenosis endoscope including a tubular retractor. (c) Approach angles in relation to the caudal endplate change dependent on the spinal segment. In the lower lumbar spine, approximately 10 to 15 degrees of distal C-arm tilt is added, while 0 to 5 degrees are typically sufficient in the upper lumbar segments.

index-level vertebral body is obtained (▶ Fig. 11.3 **a**). Based on this angle, approximately 0 to 5 degrees of caudal C-arm tilt is added in the upper lumbar segments and approximately 10 to 15 degrees in the lower lumbar segments. The goal is to center the spinous processes over the projection of the disk space (▶ Fig. 11.3 **b,c**). Choosing a too steep rostrocaudal approach angle hampers decompression of the caudal aspect of the lateral recess as the endoscope is deflected by caudal lamina. This is of particular concern in upper lumbar segments where segmental stenosis is often localized in the inferior aspect of the interlaminar window and caused by overgrowth of the sagittally oriented facet joints. Choosing an approach corridor in line with the disk space will require substantially more resection of the rostral lamina, in particular at lower lumbar levels. Once the appropriate rostrocaudal approach angle is determined, the AP fluoroscopic image should also reveal the *inferomedial edge of the rostral index-level lamina*, which is the *target area* for this approach (▶ Fig. 11.3 **d**). The skin incision is marked where the target area crosses the disk space (▶ Fig. 11.3 **d**). A small vertical skin incision is produced using a no. 11 blade. Serial dilators are advanced with small rostrocaudal movements along the AP trajectory of the fluoroscopy until *target area* can be palpated. Beveled dilators may be used to strip muscles off the lamina edge in order to *facilitate transition from palpation to visualization*. Then, the tubular retractor is advanced over the dilators until the edge

of the lamina can be palpated with the tip of the bevel (▶ Fig. 11.3 **e,f**). The open bevel of the tubular retractor should face medially to optimize retraction of the paraspinal muscles. The tubular retractor should remain in solid bone contract until the endoscope is brought to avoid soft-tissue creep.

11.4 Visualization of the Target Area

The target area is visualized first. Exposure is best accomplished by retracting overlying soft tissue with the bevel of the tubular retractor laterally and resect the tissue under tension with grasping forceps, micro-punch, and the bipolar cautery (see Chapter 9 for surgical technique). Once the inferomedial lamina edge is visualized, the exposure is extended from the base of the spinous process to the tip of inferior articular process (▶ Fig. 11.4 **a**). The lamina attachment of the yellow ligament that constitutes the *principal anatomic landmark* for the interlaminar approach might be visible at this point. Resecting bone along the inferomedial edge of the lamina with a diamond burr typically exposes the yellow ligament insertion. This maneuver is particularly useful to unambiguously visualize the principal anatomical landmark in patients with severe facet hypertrophy, scoliosis, or previous surgery (▶ Fig. 11.4 **b**).

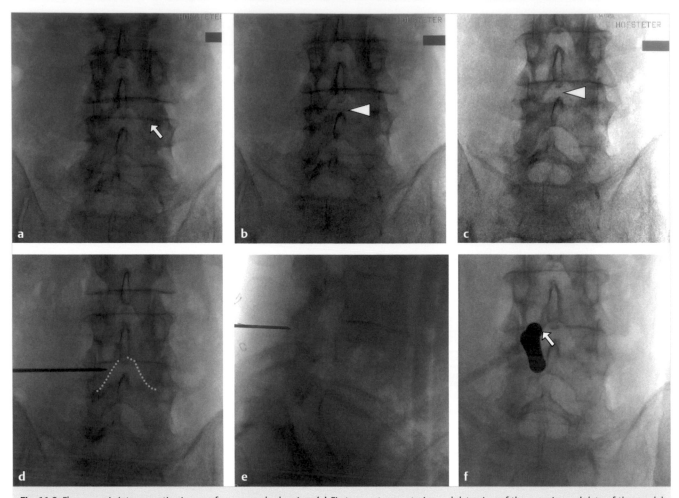

Fig. 11.3 Fluoroscopic intraoperative images for approach planning. **(a)** First, an anteroposterior endplate view of the superior endplate of the caudal spinal segment is obtained (L3/L4; *arrow*). **(b)** The addition of distal tilt to the rostrocaudal X-ray beam angle moves the projection of the interspinous process space toward the disk space (*arrowhead*). **(c)** Once the gap between the spinous processes is centered over the projection of the disk space, an ideal rostrocaudal trajectory has been determined (*arrowhead*). **(d)** The inferior edge of the superior index-level lamina (*green dotted line*) constituting the *target area* for this approach should be clearly visible. The skin incision is marked at the tip of the radiopaque object. **(e)** A lateral X-ray may be obtained to confirm the level. **(f)** Once the working tube is brought into place, an AP X-ray confirms the location of the working tube at the inferior margin of the lamina (*arrow*).

11.5 Hemilaminotomy

Using a diamond or side-biting burr, bone resection is carried out along the insertion of the yellow ligament. Bony decompression is extended rostrally until the yellow ligament thins out at the base of the spinous process and caudally to the tip of the inferior articular process (▶ Fig. 11.4 **c,d**). Bone resection along the insertion of the yellow ligament constitutes the leading edge for the bony decompression and determines the need of more superficial bone resection of the lamina or base of the spinous process. The lateral extent of the hemilaminotomy remains empirical at this stage and is completed later once the neural structures are exposed.

11.6 Enter Epidural Space

In-line resection and transgression of the yellow ligament may be carried out with the micro-punch. The punch is oriented at a right angle in relation to the yellow ligament fibers and slowly advanced with a rotational movement (for additional details on in-line soft-tissue resection, see Chapter 9; ▶ Fig. 11.5 **a**). Just prior to transgressing the ligament, a grayish blue discoloration of the ligament is commonly observed. Once the yellow ligament is opened, inflow of irrigation fluid enters the epidural space and retracts the thecal sac (▶ Fig. 11.5 **b**). Instead of a micro-punch, a blunt dissector can be used for in-line transgression of the yellow ligament. If the yellow ligament has been thinned out during the bony decompression, the opening can be widened with a Kerrison rongeur (▶ Fig. 11.5 **c**). Dense adhesions between the yellow ligament and the dura may be encountered in cases of revision surgery, extremely severe stenosis, high-grade segmental listhesis, or synovial cysts. In cases of revision surgery, additional bone may be resected to expose virgin yellow ligament and dura. In cases of severe listhesis, the dura may be partially eroded within the lateral recess. Meticulous dissection and direct continuous visualization of every Kerrison bite can help to preserve the integrity of

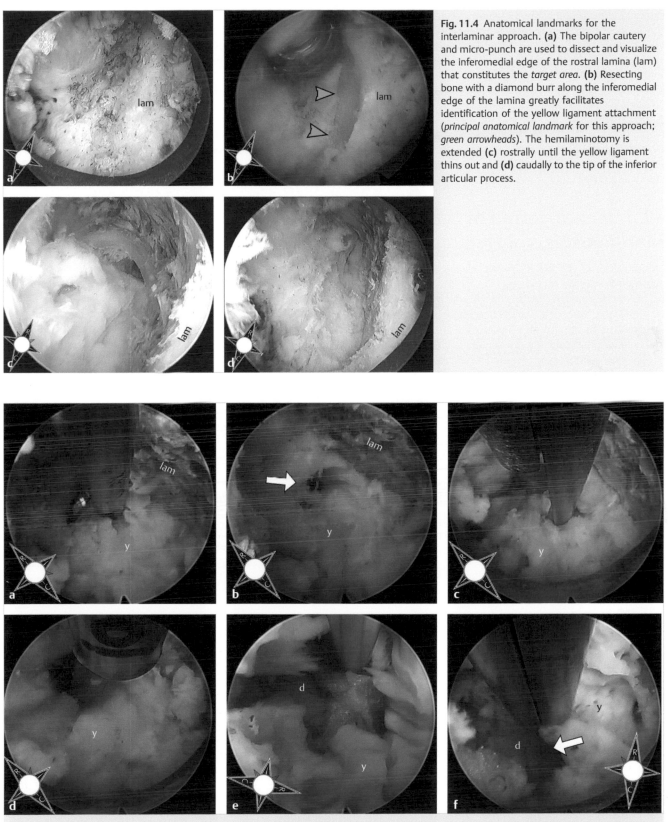

Fig. 11.4 Anatomical landmarks for the interlaminar approach. (a) The bipolar cautery and micro-punch are used to dissect and visualize the inferomedial edge of the rostral lamina (lam) that constitutes the *target area*. (b) Resecting bone with a diamond burr along the inferomedial edge of the lamina greatly facilitates identification of the yellow ligament attachment (*principal anatomical landmark* for this approach; *green arrowheads*). The hemilaminotomy is extended (c) rostrally until the yellow ligament thins out and (d) caudally to the tip of the inferior articular process.

Fig. 11.5 Enter the epidural space and identify the thecal sac. (a) The yellow ligament (y) is opened using a micro-punch oriented in a normal angle in relation to the fibers and advanced with a rotational movement. (b) Upon opening of the yellow ligament, irrigation fluid immediately retracts the epidural fat and thecal sac. (c) The opening of the yellow ligament is extended using Kerrison rongeurs. (d) The bipolar cautery is used to cauterize the inside of the yellow ligament and epidural fat tissue and vessels. (e) The dura (d) is identified. (f) Additional yellow ligament is resected until the lateral margin of the dura can be seen. Abbreviation: lam, lamina.

the dura. If no tissue plane between yellow ligament and dura can be identified, a more medial entry can be chosen, and yellow ligament resected along the midline raphe until the dura is visualized. Prior to resection of the yellow ligament, cauterization of the inside of the yellow ligament with the bipolar cautery can prevent cumbersome bleeding (▶ Fig. 11.5 **d**). Likewise, epidural fat and vessels should be cauterized prior to resection. A meticulous exposure of the dura with resection of epidural fascial layers with grasping forceps is carried out (▶ Fig. 11.5 **e**). Careful dissection and exposure of the dura is necessary for unambiguous identification of the lateral margin of the neural elements (▶ Fig. 11.5 **f**).

11.7 Identification of the Lateral Margin of Neural Elements

Identification of the lateral margin of neural elements is best accomplished in the rostral aspect of the decompression site (at or above the tip of the SAP; ▶ Fig. 11.5 **f**). Using a bipolar cautery bridging, veins and connective tissue are cauterized and ligated sharply (▶ Fig. 11.6 **a**). Turning the endoscope laterally and gently retracting the thecal sac with a blunt dissector assists with identification of the lateral margin of neural elements (▶ Fig. 11.6 **b**). In the lower lumbar segments (L4/L5 an L5/S1), the axilla of the traversing nerve root may be mistaken for the lateral margin of the neural elements. In that case, the neural elements cannot be easily medialized as they are tethered on the traversing nerve root that is physically "stuck"

in the lateral recess. Incomplete decompression of the traversing nerve root should also be suspected if the bipolar cautery directed laterally into the lateral recess leads to lower extremity muscle activation. Additional undercutting of the ipsilateral facet will release the traversing nerve root. Sufficient lateral recess decompression is confirmed by absence of tethering of the neural elements and ability to inspect the medial aspect of the caudal index-level pedicle. Once the margin of neural elements has been identified, the need and extent of additional lateral recess decompression is determined.

11.8 Lateral Recess Decompression

At this point, the hemilaminotomy is widened as necessary for decompression of the lateral recess. Maximizing off-axis reach (see Chapter 9 for details) and the use of a large-diameter diamond burr facilitates undercutting and helps to preserve the pars interarticularis. Residual yellow ligament within the lateral recess is resected using Kerrison rongeurs as well as straight and up-angled micro-punches. Resection of the medal aspect of the SAP is carried out utilizing Kerrison rongeurs or a side-cutting burr along the lateral margin of the thecal sac/traversing nerve root (▶ Fig. 11.7 **a,b**). Decompression of neural elements should extend from the tip of the SAP to the mid-portion of the caudal pedicle. In order to visualize the caudal pedicle, resection of the caudal lamina is often necessary. For this, the rostral edge of the lamina is thinned using a diamond

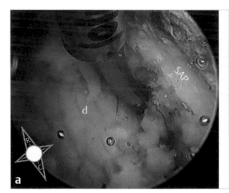
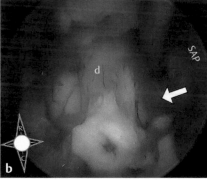

Fig. 11.6 Identification of the lateral margin of neural elements. **(a)** Directing the endoscope laterally, the bipolar is used to shrink epidural fat and to cauterize vessel lateral to the thecal sac. **(b)** The blunt dissector is used to medialize the thecal sac to identify the lateral margin of the neural elements in order to determine the extent of additional necessary lateral recess decompression.

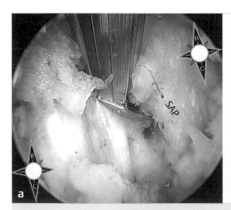
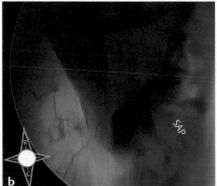
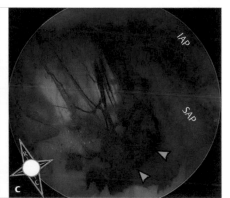

Fig. 11.7 Bony decompression of the lateral recess. The medial aspect of the superior articular process is resected using either **(a)** a Kerrison rongeur or **(b)** a side-cutting burr. **(c)** The caudal lamina overlying the traversing nerve root is resected (*arrowheads*). Abbreviations: IAP, inferior articular process; SAP, superior articular process.

burr (▶ Fig. 11.7 **c**) and residual bone and yellow ligament are resected with Kerrison rongeurs. Decompression of the caudal lamina is in particular important in cases with spondylolisthesis or large central disk protrusions in order to create sufficient space for the neural elements during physiological segmental movement.

11.9 Retraction of Neural Elements

Once bridging vessels and adhesions have been ligated, the lateral margin of the neural elements can be gently medialized using a blunt dissector (for additional details on surgical technique, see Chapter 9; ▶ Fig. 11.8 **a**). Then, the working cannula is advanced into the spinal canal with the bevel facing medially. Under continuous visualization of the neural elements, the working cannula may be rotated 180 degrees (▶ Fig. 11.8 **b**). This maneuver needs to be performed with great care as the bevel may impinge the neural elements or may lacerate the dura during the rotational maneuver. If retraction of neural elements is not easily possible, tethering of neural elements should be ruled out first. If retraction of the neural elements is still not easily possible, additional bone of the lateral recess needs to be resected.

11.10 Ventral Decompression of Neural Elements

Once the neural elements are retracted with the tubular retractor, the annulus of the disk may be inspected and defects or contained disk fragments may be visualized. In cases of

marginal osteophytes originating from the posterior endplates, ventral decompression of the traversing nerve root can be safely accomplished. This is in particular important in revision lateral recess decompressions or cases with extensive disk–osteophyte complexes. Ventral bony pathology may be resected using the diamond burr (▶ Fig. 11.8 **c**) and soft-tissue pathology such as disk annulus or posterior longitudinal ligament with the micro-punch (▶ Fig. 11.8 **d**). Once ventral pathology has been addressed, the working cannula may be withdrawn from the spinal canal. The neural elements should now be entirely decompressed, free, and pulsating. At this point, the tip of the SAP should be inspected and trimmed if necessary, and the medial wall of the caudal pedicle should be seen together with the traversing nerve root with perineural fat when entering into the foraminal zone (▶ Fig. 11.9). This concludes decompression of the lateral recess.

11.11 Pearls and Pitfalls

- The skin incision should not be too large in order to avoid leakage of irrigation fluid and inability to build up appropriate fluid pressure.
- Inability to transition from radiographic localization of the target area to palpation. Difficulties at this stage may be due to an inadequate AP X-ray or a surgical approach trajectory not in line with the AP X-ray. Taking a look at the orientation of the endoscope in relation to the C-arm often helps.
- Direct approach onto the yellow ligament at L5/S1. Experienced surgeons may dock on the yellow ligament directly omitting palpation of inferomedial lamina edge. In these cases, lateral fluoroscopic images may help confirm appropriate depth. Blind penetration of the yellow ligament is not advised as it could lead to damage of neural structures.

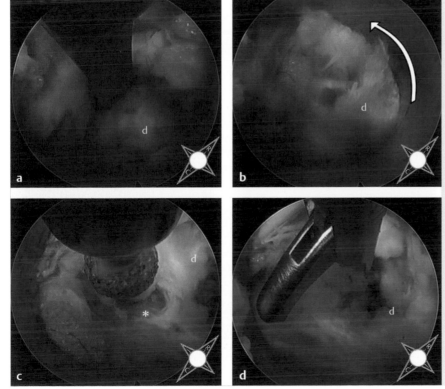

Fig. 11.8 Retraction and ventral decompression of neural elements. **(a)** The lateral margin of the neural elements is gently medialized using the blunt dissector. **(b)** The working cannula is advanced into the spinal canal and rotated 180 degrees to retract the neural elements. **(c)** An osteophyte (*asterisk*) originating from the posterior aspect of the inferior endplate is resected using a diamond burr. **(d)** Protruding annulus is resected using the micro-punch. Abbreviation: d, disk.

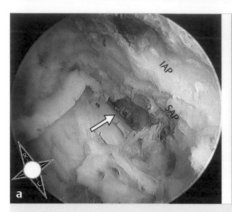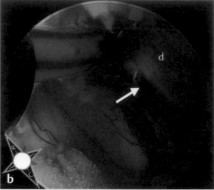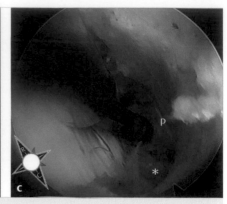

Fig. 11.9 Confirmation of adequate lateral recess decompression. **(a)** The lateral margin of the neural elements (*arrow*) is seen from the tip of the superior articular process to the mid-portion of the caudal pedicle. **(b)** Adequate decompression of neural elements is confirmed at the level of the intervertebral disk (d). **(c)** The caudal pedicle (p) is seen and the traversing nerve root is noted to be covered by perineural fat (*asterisk*). Abbreviations: IAP, inferior articular process; SAP, superior articular process.

- Bone bleeding can be tedious to control, in particular small arterial bleeders in the sclerotic bone underlying degenerated facet joints. They may be addressed with the bipolar cautery, high-speed diamond drill bit, or tamponaded with a blunt dissector or Kerrison rongeur. Injection of thrombin into the endoscope may help. See Chapter 8 for additional strategies to manage intraoperative bleeding.
- Inability to identify the yellow ligament attachment following bone removal. Typically, the bone work is done either too medial within the base of the spinous process or too lateral in the facet joint. Obtain AP and lateral X-rays to get reoriented. The lamina insertion of the yellow ligament is the principal anatomical landmark for the bony decompression during the interlaminar approach, and inability to unambiguously localize it constitutes an absolute need to halt the procedure. Repeat fluoroscopic imaging, and check approach trajectory, palpation of the inferomedial edge of the lamina, and X-ray confirmation of the tip of the instrument.
- Inability to identify dura after transgressing the yellow ligament. The entry into the canal might be too lateral or in the axilla of the nerve root, in particular at L5/S1. In upper spinal segments, the inside of the contralateral yellow ligament can be mistaken for the thecal sac. Good preparation of the thecal sac and attention to detail such as orientation of the endoscope, relation to the bony landmarks, and pulsations of the thecal sac help unambiguously identify the neural elements.

- The lateral margin of the neural element cannot be visualized. Typically, additional resection of the medial facet is necessary. The lateral margin is easiest identified rostral to the SAP.
- Access to the medial portion of the SAP can be facilitated by gently retracting the inferior articular process with the tubular retractor. This maneuver should only be carried out very gently and avoided in patients with osteoporosis as it can fracture the inferior articular process.
- Lateral margin of the neural elements cannot easily be medialized. This is typically the case when the thecal sac is medialized in the axilla. The traversing nerve root might be physically "stuck" in the lateral recess. This is commonly observed at L4/L5 and L5/S1. More undercutting of the ipsilateral facet is necessary until the traversing nerve root is decompressed and released.
- Scar tissues/disk herniation obscuring the lateral margin. Increase the rostral and caudal exposure and apply gentle traction to the thecal sac with the blunt dissector. This typically reveals the interface between the dura and the scar tissue.
- In the cases with spondylolisthesis, the entire rostrocaudal extent of the inferior articular process needs to be undercut as residual bone spurs may cause entrapment of the lateral recess during translational movement.

12 Interlaminar Endoscopic Lumbar Diskectomy

Lynn McGrath and Christoph P. Hofstetter

12.1 Case Example

A 60-year-old woman presents with a 6-month history of left lower extremity radicular pain (7/10 in severity) radiating into her posterior calf. On examination, the patient has a left missing ankle reflex. Preoperative MRI reveals a left L5/S1 disk protrusion without migration and impingement of the left traversing S1 nerve root (▶ Fig. 12.1). *The procedure performed was left interlaminar endoscopic L5/S1 diskectomy.* One year after the procedure, the patient's radiculopathy has resolved and she has minimal residual numbness.

12.2 Indications

The interlaminar endoscopic approach is well suited for resection of subarticular disk herniations, in particular in the lower lumbar segments. At L5/S1, minimal or no bony resection is necessary to approach the pathology. For subarticular disk herniations at L4/L5, a medial facetectomy is typically necessary to gain access to the pathology. In upper lumbar segments, the interlaminar approach is less ideal for diskectomies given the narrow pedicle-to-pedicle distance and sagittally oriented facet joints. The interlaminar approach is well suited for rostrally or caudally migrated disk herniations since pathology can be reached by adjusting the rostrocaudal approach angle and/or additional lamina resection. The interlaminar approach for disk herniations is particularly useful in cases of subarticular disk herniations and concomitant lateral recess stenosis in lower lumbar spine L4/L5 and L5/S1. The following factors favor the interlaminar approach:

- Lower lumbar segment (L4/L5 or L5/S1).
- Migrated disk fragments.
- Concomitant ipsilateral recess stenosis (see Chapter 11).
- Need for additional central or contralateral decompression (see Chapters 13 and 14).

See Chapter 6 for operating room setup and patient positioning.

12.3 Approach

As with other interlaminar approaches, the approach angle is extremely important. Initially, an endplate view of the caudal vertebral body is obtained on anteroposterior (AP) fluoroscopy. For nonmigrated disk herniations, the interlaminar window is optimized by adding approximately 0 to 5 degrees of distal C-arm tilt in the upper lumbar segments and approximately 10 to 15 degrees in the lower lumbar segments (▶ Fig. 12.2 **a,d,g**). Caudally migrated disk herniations can be reached using less distal C-arm tilt (▶ Fig. 12.2 **b,e,h**). However, this may require a medial facetectomy and resection of the superior portion of the caudal lamina (see Chapter 11). Rostrally migrated disk fragments may be approached with a steeper rostrocaudal angulation (▶ Fig. 12.2 **c,f,i**). However, if the approach angle is too steep, the working tube may be deflected by the caudal index-level lamina, in particular in patients with a steep sacral slope. In any case, the approach angle chosen should allow for inspection of the disk annulus for annular tears and loose contained disk fragments. A vertical skin incision is marked where the determined rostrocaudal trajectory intersects with the *inferomedial edge of the rostral index-level lamina (target area).* For operations at L5/S1, the *interlaminar window* may serve as *target area.*

12.3.1 Tissue Dilation and Placement of Working Tube

Once the skin incision is marked, a small vertical skin and thoracolumbar fascia incision is produced using a no. 11 blade. The first trocar is advanced with small rostrocaudal movements along the AP trajectory of the fluoroscopy until the edge of the lamina or the yellow ligament are reached. In case of the latter, a lateral X-ray should be obtained to confirm appropriate depth of the instruments as blind penetration of the yellow ligament is not advised. Then, serial dilators are brought in with the open bevel facing medially. These dilators may be used to dissect off muscle tissue from the bony edges, which greatly facilitates the

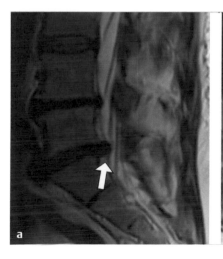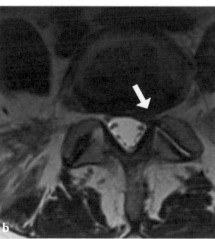

Fig. 12.1 Preoperative MRI depicting a nonmigrated left L5/S1 disk herniation. **(a)** Arrow indicates the protruding disk in a sagittal T2-weighted MRI. **(b)** An axial image reveals the impingement of the left traversing S1 nerve root (*arrow*).

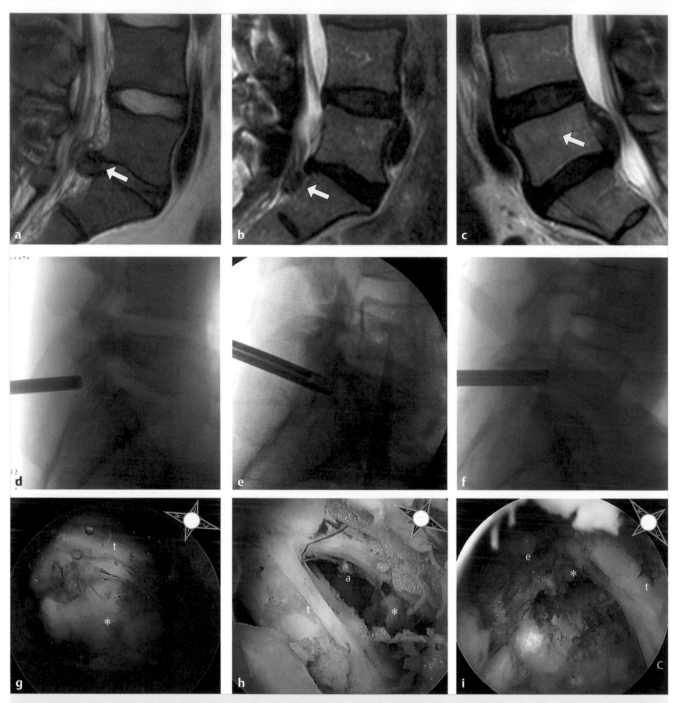

Fig. 12.2 Sagittal T2-weighted MRI revealing **(a)** nonmigrated, **(b)** caudally migrated, and **(c)** rostrally migrated disk fragments. **(d)** For a nonmigrated L5/S1 herniation, the rostrocaudal angulation of the working cannula is approximately 20 degrees in relation to the S1 endplate. **(e)** For distally migrated fragments, the working cannula is in line with the S1 endplate and **(f)** for rostrally migrated fragments, it is approximately 35 degrees. Intraoperative views of **(g)** a nondisplaced disk fragment (*asterisk*), **(h)** caudally migrated fragment (*asterisk*), and **(i)** rostrally migrated fragment (*asterisks*). (Abbreviations: t, traversing nerve root; a, axilla; e, exiting nerve root.)

transition from palpation to visualization. Finally, the working tube is brought in with the bevel facing medially, the dilators are withdrawn, and the endoscope is introduced.

12.3.2 Visualization of the Target Area

Using the pituitary rongeur and the bipolar cautery, the paraspinal muscle overlying the yellow ligament is resected.

Typically, a thin layer of fat is encountered superficial to the yellow ligament (▶ Fig. 12.3 **a**). Once the yellow ligament is reached, the working cannula is utilized to retract muscle tissue. In cases that require some degree of hemilaminotomy (typically any level above L5/S1), visualization of the yellow ligament may be facilitated by drilling along the inferomedial edge of the lamina with a diamond burr (▶ Fig. 12.3 **b**).

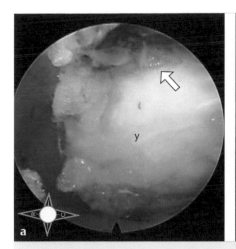 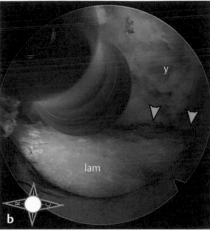 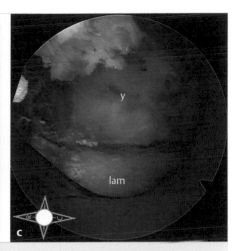

Fig. 12.3 Identification of the yellow ligament (*principal anatomical landmark*). Initial view of the yellow ligament (y) during a L5/S1 approach via the large interlaminar window. (**a**) Note the small layer of fat tissue between the paraspinal muscle tissue and the yellow ligament (*arrow*). (**b**) The attachment of the yellow ligament (*green arrowheads*) is identified by resecting bone along the inferomedial aspect of the rostral lamina (lam) using a diamond burr. (**c**) The yellow ligament is exposed within the area of the hemilaminotomy.

12.3.3 Hemilaminotomy

In lumbar segments above L5/S1, a small hemilaminotomy is performed by resecting bone along lamina attachment of the yellow ligament a using a diamond burr (▶ Fig. 12.3 **c**; for surgical technique, see Chapter 11). Additional resection of rostral or caudal lamina may be carried out to gain access to migrated disk fragments. The extent of the hemilaminotomy remains empirical at this stage and is completed later together with a lateral recess decompression if necessary, once the lateral margin of the neural structures has been determined.

12.4 Enter Epidural Space

For the interlaminar endoscopic diskectomy, the yellow ligament serves as the *principal anatomical landmark* for safe identification of the epidural space and neural elements. There are various techniques to safely transgress the yellow ligament. A micro-punch oriented at a right angle to the ligament fibers is slowly advanced with rotational and rostrocaudal movements (▶ Fig. 12.4 **a**). The resection area is widened by placing the straight jaw of the micro-punch into the defect and resecting the edge with the articulating jaw (▶ Fig. 12.4 **b**). The bevel of the tubular retractor can be utilized retract the incised portion of the yellow ligament to facilitate dissection. Just prior to transgressing the ligament, a grayish blue discoloration of the ligament can me observed (▶ Fig. 12.4 **c**). The ligament should first be transgressed with the open jaw of the micro-punch utilizing it like a Penfield dissector no. 4. Once the yellow ligament is opened, inflow of irrigation fluid immediately retracts the epidural fat and thecal sac. Following coagulation of the inside of the yellow ligament with the bipolar cautery to prevent bleeding, the opening is widened using the Kerrison rongeur (▶ Fig. 12.4 **d**). For additional technical details regarding the in-line transgression of the yellow ligament, see Chapter 9.

12.4.1 Identify Lateral Margin of Neural Elements

Epidural fat, vessels, and fascial layers are thoroughly dissected off the thecal sac. Exposure of the dural surface is essential for identification of the interface between the neural elements and disk herniations (▶ Fig. 12.5 **a**). This is of particular importance in cases of large scarred-in disk fragments or revision diskectomies. Vessels and adhesions bridging to the lateral margin of the neural elements are coagulated with the bipolar cautery and sharply ligated. Then, the neural elements are gently mobilized using the blunt dissector (▶ Fig. 12.5 **b**). At this point, a first visual assessment of the disk herniation is possible.

12.4.2 Resection of Disk Sequester

In case of large disk sequesters underneath/medial to the traversing nerve root, it may be necessary to partially retrieve the sequester prior to medialization of the nerve root. Forceful medialization of the nerve root with the working tube against the disk sequester may lead to impingement and damage of the nerve root. Therefore, it is advisable to remove loose disk sequesters prior to medialization of the neural elements. First, the working tube may be gently advanced into the spinal canal with the open bevel facing medially to allow for partial retraction of the neural elements. Once visualized, the disk sequester may be dissected off the neural elements and mobilized using the blunt dissector and/or the bipolar cautery. Using up-angled cup forceps, loose disk fragments may be retrieved at the lateral margin of the neural elements or via the axilla (▶ Fig. 12.5 **c–f**). Retrieving fragment with an alligator maneuver under continuous direct visualization helps avoid laceration of the thecal sac.

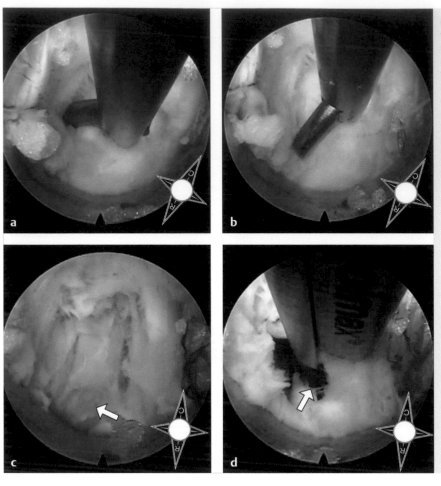

Fig. 12.4 Enter the epidural space. **(a)** In order to transgress the yellow ligament, the micro-punch is oriented at a right angle to the fibers and then advanced with a rotational movement. The yellow ligament is first transgressed with the leading edge of the open articulating jaw. **(b)** The opening is enlarged using the micro-punch. **(c)** A grayish discoloration of the yellow ligament is noted prior to transgression (*arrow*). Once the yellow ligament is opened, the irrigation fluid enlarges the epidural space (*arrow*). **(d)** The opening of the yellow ligament is enlarged using a Kerrison rongeur.

12.4.3 Retraction of Neural Elements

Once loose disk fragments have been retrieved, the traversing root is mobilized using a blunt dissector. For retraction of the neural elements, the blunt dissector may be left in place while the working tube with the open bevel facing medially is advanced into the spinal canal (▶ Fig. 12.5 **g**). Applying downward pressure, the working tube is rotated 180 degrees in order to achieve complete retraction and protection of the neural elements (▶ Fig. 12.5 **h,i**). There should be only minimal resistance to retraction of the neural elements. If retraction is tedious and the edge of the working cannula impinges the edge of the neural elements, it is advised to halt the maneuver and to rule out residual disk sequesters or a location of the working cannula within the axilla of the traversing nerve root. If retraction of neural elements remains tedious, additional bone resection of the medial facet should be considered.

12.4.4 Resection of Residual Disk Fragments and Exploration of the Annular Defect

With the neural elements retracted, the annular defect is identified (▶ Fig. 12.6 **a**). Loose disk fragments are retrieved with grasping forceps. The edges of the remaining disk are trimmed

using a micro-punch and the surface of the remaining disk may be coagulated using the bipolar cautery (▶ Fig. 12.6 **b**). The protruding portions of the disk annulus may be resected using the micro-punch. In case of a protruding osteophyte–disk complex, marginal osteophytes originating from the posterior endplates may be resected using the diamond burr. Once completed, the tubular retractor is withdrawn from the spinal canal and adequate decompression of the traversing nerve root is visually confirmed.

12.5 Pearls and Pitfalls

- Approach angle: For pathology rostral to the disk space, a steeper approach angle may be necessary. However, choosing a too steep approach angle makes entry into the disk space for resection of contained disk fragments difficult. Moreover, at L5/S1 a steep approach angle can interfere with adequate lateral recess decompression, in particular in patients with a steep sacral slope, since the endoscope is deflected by the S1 lamina. On the contrary, a too flat approach angle in line with the endplate view may lead to the need for an extensive hemilaminotomy, increased procedure time, and possible weakening of the pars interarticularis.
- Difficulty to transition from radiographic depiction of the target area (either inferomedial edge of the lamina or

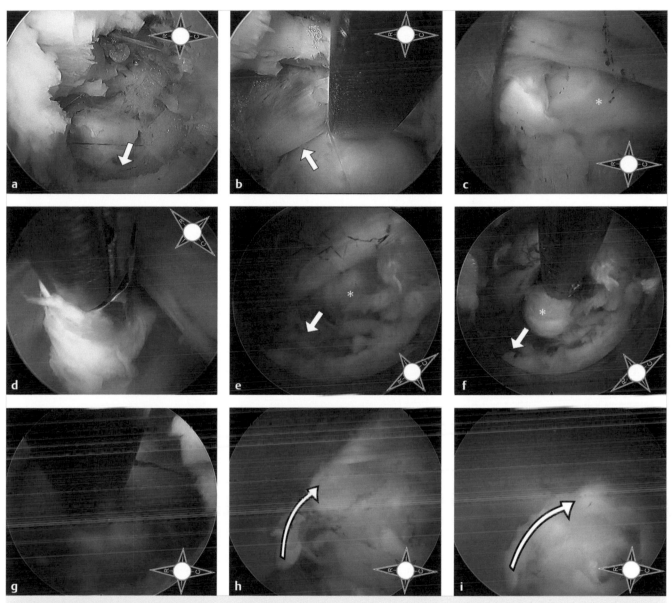

Fig. 12.5 Identification of the lateral margin of neural elements, resection of disk sequesters, and retraction of neural elements. **(a)** The lateral margin of the neural elements (*arrow*) is identified in the superior portion of the operative field. **(b)** The neural elements (*arrow*) are gently medialized using a blunt dissector. **(c,d)** In case of a large disk fragment ventral to the traversing nerve root (*arrow*), the disk sequesters (*asterisk*) may be retrieved using grasping forceps using rotational movement. **(e,f)** In case of a large disk fragment (*asterisk*) at L5/S1, the disk sequester might be retrieved via the axilla of the traversing nerve root (*arrow*). **(g)** Once the traversing nerve root is partially decompressed, the traversing nerve root is mobilized using the blunt dissector and the tubular working sleeve is advanced into the spinal canal with the bevel facing medially. **(h,i)** The nerve root is then retracted medially by rotating the working sleeve carefully 180 degrees maintaining visualization of the traversing nerve root in order to avoid impingement of this neural structure during this maneuver.

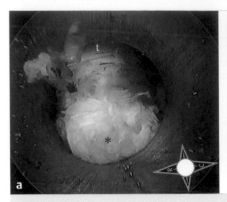 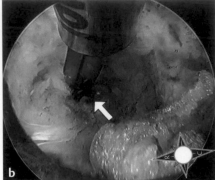 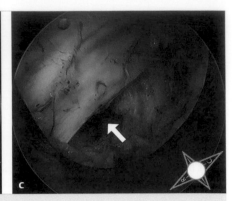

Fig. 12.6 Resection of contained disk fragments. **(a)** With the neural elements retracted, loose disk fragments (*asterisk*) are retrieved via the annular defect using grasping forceps. **(b)** Once all loose fragments are removed, the surface of the remaining disk and the annulus are coagulated (*arrow points* at the annular defect). **(c)** The decompressed traversing nerve root is inspected following complete decompression (*arrow points* at the annular defect).

interlaminar window) to palpation with the trocar may be due to an inadequate AP X-ray or an approach trajectory not in line with the X-ray. Taking a look at the orientation of the trocar in relation to the C-arm often helps.
- Inferomedial edge of the lamina was palpated with the trocar, dilators, and bevel of the tubular retractor; however, once the scope is brought in, it is not visible. Possible reasons include the following:
  ○ Endoscope not in line with the X-ray. Remedy: check orientation of C-arm and make sure that the endoscope is aligned.
- Working tube has been expulsed—reestablish solid contact with the bony edge and maintain contact during introduction of endoscope.
- Large overgrown facet joint: Dissect part of the joint and try to palpate bony edge with tools via the working channel and resect bone along the inferomedial lamina to detect yellow

ligament attachment. Obtain AP and lateral X-rays to confirm appropriate location.
- Direct approach onto the yellow ligament at L5/S1: Experienced surgeons may dock on the yellow ligament directly omitting identification of the bony attachment of the yellow ligament. However, palpating the inferior edge of the lamina can help assess the depth of the instruments and can sometimes avoid the need for lateral X-rays.
- Difficulties mobilizing the lateral margin of the neural elements. Rule out adhesions, bridging vessels, or disk fragments. Moreover, confirm that medialization is not attempted within the axilla of the traversing nerve root. In that case, the tethering nerve can typically be seen in the rostral part of the surgical field and use of the bipolar cautery to coagulate bridging vessels irritates the traversing nerve root within the lateral recess.
- The degree of resection of disk material contained in the disk space remains controversial.

13 Interlaminar Contralateral Endoscopic Lumbar Foraminotomy

Christoph P. Hofstetter

13.1 Case Example

A 49-year-old woman presents with a 1-year history of left lower extremity radicular pain. The pain radiates from her lower back, to the left buttock, lateral thigh, and lateral calf. The patient rates the pain as 9.5 out of 10 in severity. After standing or walking for more than 10 minutes, her entire left leg turns numb and give out. On physical examination, the patient is neurologically intact. An MRI (▶ Fig. 13.1 **a,b**) of the patient's lumbar spine revealed severe left L5/S1 foraminal stenosis mainly due to vertical foraminal stenosis (foraminal height 12 mm) and subluxation of the S1 superior articular process (SAP). The patient underwent an *interlaminar contralateral endoscopic left L5/S1 foraminotomy*. Ten months after surgery, the patient is neurologically intact. The patient rates her leg pain as 2/10.

13.2 Indications

Interlaminar contralateral endoscopic foraminotomies may be considered for the treatment of symptomatic lumbar foraminal stenosis mainly at L5/S1. The approach corridor requires a laminotomy and contralateral medial facetectomy, which is more labor intensive compared to an ipsilateral transforaminal approaches. Moreover, given the narrow working corridor, less bony foraminal decompression can be achieved, in particular within the lateral aspect of the foramen compared to a transforaminal approach. However, the interlaminar contralateral endoscopic approach constitutes a valuable alternative for certain selected situations: first, in patients with high iliac crests in whom an L5/S1 transforaminal approach is difficult or not feasible. Second, in patients who also require decompression of neural elements within the spinal canal, this procedure may be added for decompression of the contralateral exiting nerve root. The interlaminar contralateral approach allows effective decompression of the medial aspect of the foramen. Appropri-

ate indications include foraminal stenosis caused by SAP hypertrophy, yellow ligament hypertrophy, bony fragments of the SAP, or synovial cysts. The interlaminar contralateral endoscopic approach is not well suited for treatment of vertical foraminal stenosis since resection of the superior portion of the caudal index pedicle is cumbersome and inefficient. In particular, interlaminar contralateral decompression of vertical foraminal stenosis in the setting of segmental coronal deformity provides typically only transient symptomatic relief and the authors consider this pathology a relative contraindication for direct decompression surgery. Patients with vertical foraminal stenosis (pedicle-to-pedicle foraminal height of < 10 mm) due to segmental coronal deformity may be better candidates for indirect decompression utilizing an interbody graft and segmental arthrodesis.

13.3 Approach

Given that the space between the index-level spinous processes is utilized as the surgical corridor to the contralateral foramen, precise determination of the rostrocaudal approach angle is important. An endplate view of the caudal vertebral body is obtained on anteroposterior (AP) fluoroscopy. Then, approximately 20 to 30 degrees of kyphosis of the C-arm are added until the skin entry point, the gap between interspinous processes, and the superior portion of the contralateral SAP line up (▶ Fig. 13.2 **a**). The rostrocaudal approach angle is significantly steeper compared to a typical approach for central or lateral recess decompression surgeries. If the approach angle is not steep enough, the contralateral foramen is difficult to reach since the approach corridor is blocked by the base of the spinous process and the contralateral lamina. Even additional resection of the base of the spinous process and lamina is of only limited value since the narrow bony corridor limits the amount of foraminal decompression that can be achieved (▶ Fig. 13.2 **b**). A small vertical skin incision is made where a

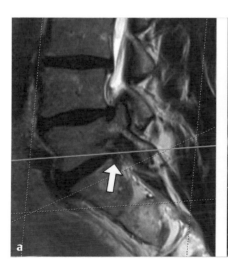 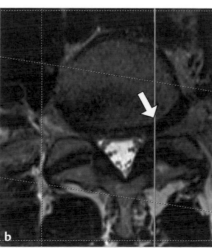

Fig. 13.1 MRI depicts L5/S1 foraminal stenosis in a young female. **(a)** Sagittal T2-weighted images reveal impingement of the exiting L5 nerve root by a combination of foraminal height loss, disk bulge, and subluxation of the S1 superior articular process (*arrow*). **(b)** The axial T2-weighted MRI shows a broad-based disk bulge contributing to the foraminal stenosis (*arrow*).

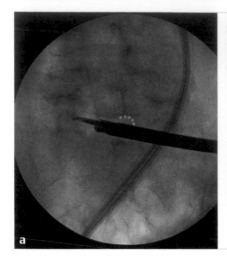
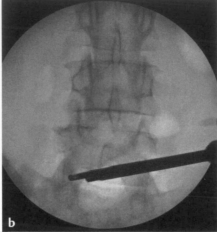

Fig. 13.2 Intraoperative fluoroscopic image showing (a) an ideal and (b) a suboptimal approach angle. The ideal approach angle allows for a working corridor between the L5 and S1 spinous processes. The target area (inferior lamina edge at the spinolaminar junction) is marked with a *dotted green line*. (b) In this case, an approach corridor with too little kyphotic angulation has been chosen. This requires extensive resection of lamina and the base of the spinous process and greatly narrows the approach corridor towards the target.

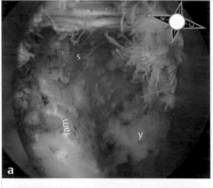
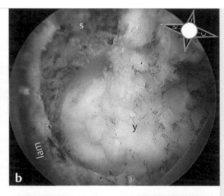
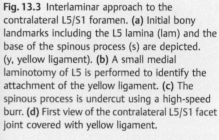

Fig. 13.3 Interlaminar approach to the contralateral L5/S1 foramen. (a) Initial bony landmarks including the L5 lamina (lam) and the base of the spinous process (s) are depicted. (y, yellow ligament). (b) A small medial laminotomy of L5 is performed to identify the attachment of the yellow ligament. (c) The spinous process is undercut using a high-speed burr. (d) First view of the contralateral L5/S1 facet joint covered with yellow ligament.

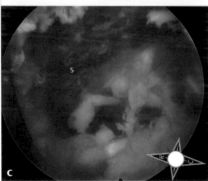
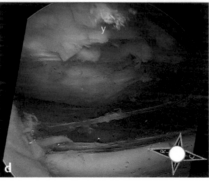

line between the superior portion of contralateral SAP and interspinous gap crosses the lateral aspect of the facet joint. Serial dilators are advanced along the rostrocaudal plane of the AP X-ray aiming slightly medially with small rostrocaudal movements toward the inferior lamina edge at the spinolaminar junction (*target area*). Beveled dilators may be used to strip muscles off the lamina edge in order to facilitate the transition from palpation to visualization. Attention should be paid to maintain solid contact with the edge of the lamina. Following the serial dilation, the working tube is placed with the bevel facing medially. At this point, the endoscope is introduced.

13.4 Identify Bony Landmarks

The first endoscopic view often reveals paraspinal muscle tissue and ideally some bony surface of the lamina, where muscle was detached by the serial dilators. If no bony surface is seen, the working sleeve should be used to palpate the lamina edge and to retract overlying soft tissue. Soft tissue is resected using the bipolar cautery and the micro-punch until the edge of the lamina in the target area becomes visible (▶ Fig. 13.3 **a**).

13.5 Laminotomy

Using a diamond or side-cutting burr, a laminotomy is initiated along the inferior aspect of the lamina along the insertion of the yellow ligament. The base of the spinous process is undercut along the insertion of the yellow ligament (▶ Fig. 13.3 **b**). Undercutting of the base of the spinous process is continued until the contralateral lamina becomes visible. Paying close attention to the transition of cancellous bone found in the base of the spinous process to cortical bone seen in the contralateral

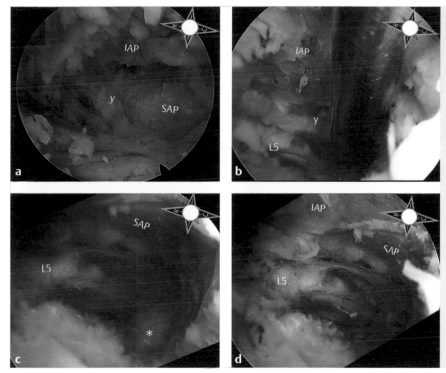

Fig. 13.4 Decompression of the contralateral L5/ S1 foramen. Following resection of the yellow ligament, the S1 superior articular process (SAP; *principal anatomical landmark*) is seen. **(a)** Note that the exiting L5 nerve root is still covered and compressed by the yellow ligament (y) attached to the tip of the SAP. Following resection of the SAP, the exiting L5 nerve root is seen. **(b)** The foraminal yellow ligament (y) contributes to the foraminal stenosis. **(c)** A foraminal disk herniation (*asterisk*) is seen and resected using pituitary rongeurs. **(d)** The circumferentially decompressed L5 nerve root is seen in the L5/S1 foramen. Abbreviation: IAP, inferior articular process.

lamina helps recognize the transition to the contralateral side (▶ Fig. 13.3 **c**). Once the attachment of yellow ligament on the inside of the contralateral lamina is identified, the yellow ligament can be stripped off the ventral lamina using a sharp dissector. This maneuver reveals the angulation of the contralateral lamina and thus defines the direction of the bony working corridor toward the contralateral foramen. Moreover, stripping off yellow ligament facilitates resection using the grasping forceps or Kerrison rongeur.

13.6 Enter Epidural Space

Entering the epidural space is accomplished by transgressing the yellow ligament using a micro-punch and Kerrison rongeurs. Prior to resection of the yellow ligament cauterization of the inside of the yellow ligament with the bipolar cautery can minimize cumbersome bleeding. Likewise, epidural fat and vessels should be cauterized prior to resection. The epidural space between the dura and the inside of the yellow ligament is followed to the contralateral facet joint. Frequently, the bulging facet joint covered with the yellow ligament can be seen (▶ Fig. 13.3 **d**).

13.7 Contralateral Recess Decompression

The yellow ligament overlying the contralateral facet joint is resected using Kerrison rongeurs. The contralateral *SAP*, which serves as the *principal anatomical landmark* for this approach, is exposed from the tip to the mid-portion of the caudal pedicle. A protected side-cutting burr may be utilized to undercut the SAP in order to decompress the contralateral recess. Using a

blunt dissector, the contralateral foramen, disk, and pedicle may be palpated and visualized. The contralateral traversing nerve root is visualized, decompressed, and mobilized.

13.8 Contralateral Foraminotomy

The yellow ligament attached to the ventral aspect of the SAP is gently mobilized using a sharp dissector and left in place as it may serve as a protective layer during the bony decompression of the exiting nerve root (▶ Fig. 13.4 **a**). Bony foraminal decompression is initiated along the ventral portion of the SAP. This may be accomplished with side-cutting burs and Kerrison rongeurs. Frequently, additional undercutting of the spinous process and the contralateral lamina is necessary to allow for sufficient bony decompression of the foramen. Use of deflecting/articulating burrs is very useful to maximize foraminal bony decompression, in particular in the lateral portion of the foramen. The goal is to identify and resect the tip of the SAP and to achieve bony foraminal decompression extending to the lateral aspect of the S1 pedicle (▶ Fig. 13.4 **b**). In addition to resection of the SAP, the superior portion of the S1 pedicle and marginal osteophytes originating from the posterior index-level endplates may be resected. During foraminal bony decompression, significant arterial bleeding can be encountered from perineural vessels and intraforaminal vessels (see Chapter 7 for further anatomical details). Bleeding can be cumbersome since visualization of the bleeder is often difficult, and extensive use of the bipolar cautery adjacent to the exiting nerve root may contribute to postoperative paresthesias. Once the bony decompression has been completed, foraminal yellow ligament may be resected using the up-angled micro-punch and Kerrison rongeur. At this point, foraminal disk herniations may be resected using the micro-punch and grasping forceps (▶ Fig. 13.4 **c**).

Upon completion of the foraminal decompression, the exiting nerve root is decompressed spanning from the rostral pedicle to the lateral aspect of the caudal pedicle, which may be confirmed with an intraoperative X-ray (▶ Fig. 13.4 **d**).

13.9 Pearls and Pitfalls

- If the rostrocaudal approach angle is not steep enough and the surgical corridor is obstructed by the base of the spinous process, the best is to produce a new skin incision more caudally.

- In patients with large interlaminar window, defining the inferior aspect of the rostral lamina may not be necessary. The contralateral foramen may be approached dissecting along the rostral edge of the inferior lamina to the contralateral SAP.
- Arterial bleeding from perineural vessels: Transiently increase the irrigation pressure, visualize the bleeding vessel, compress the vessel with the tip of the bipolar, and cauterize while applying gentle pressure. Use only bursts of cauterization to avoid heat buildup given the proximity of the nerve root and its dorsal root ganglion.

14 Lumbar Endoscopic Unilateral Laminotomy for Bilateral Decompression

Saqib Hasan and Christoph P. Hofstetter

14.1 Case Example

A 74-year-old woman presents with a 9-year history of lower back pain and lower extremity neurogenic claudication. The patient rates her back pain as 7/10 and the lower extremity pain as 5/10 in severity. The symptoms have progressed despite extensive physical therapy and five epidural steroid injections. In the months prior to presentation, the patient had developed weakness of her right lower extremity with right foot dorsiflexion (4/5) and right plantar flexion (2/5) weakness. Preoperative MRI revealed severe L4/L5 spinal stenosis with a grade 1 anterolisthesis (▶ Fig. 14.1). A flexion/extension X-ray confirmed stability of the L4/L5 motion segment with translational and rotational segmental motion within physiological range. *The procedure performed was right L4/L5 endoscopic unilateral laminotomy for bilateral decompression (ULBD).* After 1-year follow-up, the patient is neurologically intact. The patient rates her back pain as 2/10 and her lower extremity pain as 0/10.

14.2 Indications

Lumbar endoscopic ULBD allows for effective decompression of central and bilateral recess stenosis in patients presenting with primarily leg or buttock symptoms with neurogenic claudication. Surgical indications are consistent with open or minimally invasive laminectomies. Similar to the minimally invasive tubular technique, the full-endoscopic technique allows for decompression of the neural elements primarily at the level of the disk–facet joint complex. Thus, degenerative lumbar spinal stenosis is an appropriate indication for this procedure. In contrast, endoscopic ULBD may be less effective to achieve sufficient decompression in cases of epidural hematomas, lipomatosis, or infectious phlegmon as these pathologies are typically not confined to the disk–facet joint complex but often expand beyond these structures. Endoscopic ULBD may be combined with resection of synovial cysts, diskectomies (see Chapter 12),

and contralateral foraminotomies (see Chapter 13). Full-endoscopic technique is in particular advantageous compared to open and MIS technique for spinal decompression in obese patients, since a thick subcutaneous fat pannus neither requires additional exposure nor affects the lengths of working corridor or the quality of illumination/visualization. Grade 1 spondylolisthesis is not a contraindication as long as there is no dynamic instability on flexion/extension X-rays or vertical foraminal stenosis. Contraindications to lumbar endoscopic unilateral laminotomies for bilateral decompression include grade 2 spondylolisthesis, isthmic spondylolysis, significant lateral listhesis, or significant scoliosis (sagittal vertical axis [SVA] > 6 cm; lumbar lordosis–pelvic incidence (LL-PI) mismatch > 10 degrees; coronal Cobb > 20).

14.3 Approach

Determination of an optimal rostrocaudal approach angle for endoscopic ULBD is of extreme importance. Precise determination of the approach angle enlarges the interlaminar window and greatly reduces the need for bone removal and operative time. Moreover, an optimized approach angle helps spare the pars interarticularis, as the spinal canal is approached via the inferior portion of the lamina. An optimal approach angle needs to provide access to spinal canal spanning from the tip of the superior articular process (SAP) to the mid-portion of the pedicle of the caudal index-level, which constitutes the desired rostrocaudal extent of decompression. Moreover, an optimal approach angle allows for access to the contralateral recess via the gap between the index-level spinous processes. Choosing a too steep approach trajectory interferes with access to the caudal aspect of the contralateral recess as the endoscope is deflected by the caudal spinous process. Choosing a too flat approach trajectory requires more extensive undercutting of the spinous process and hinders efficient contralateral decompression. For intraoperative determination of the rostrocaudal

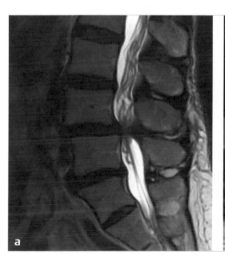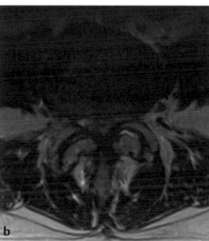

Fig. 14.1 Preoperative **(a)** sagittal and axial **(b)** T2-weighted MRI depicts severe stenosis and grade 1 anterolisthesis at L4/L5. Hypertrophy of the cauda equina nerve roots is seen on the sagittal image. No CSF is seen between the nerve roots on the axial image confirming severe central and bilateral lateral recess stenosis.

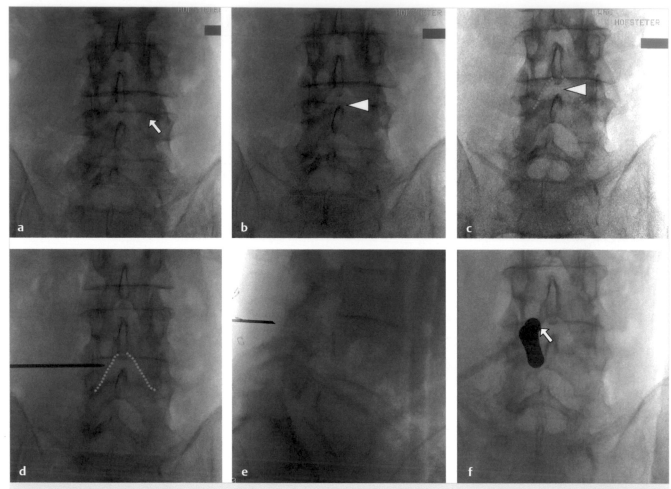

Fig. 14.2 Anteroposterior (AP) fluoroscopic intraoperative images for approach planning. **(a)** First, an AP endplate view of the L4 level is obtained (*arrow*). **(b)** The addition of caudal tilt to the X-ray beam angle moves the projection of the interspinous process space toward the disk space (*arrowhead*). **(c)** Increasing the distal C-arm tilt centers the interspinous process space onto the disk space. The ideal rostrocaudal approach trajectory has been determined (*arrowhead*). The *green dotted line* indicates the inferomedial edge of the lamina (*target area*). **(d)** The skin incision is marked where the edge of the lamina crosses the disk center. **(e)** A lateral X-ray may be obtained to confirm the level. **(f)** Once the working tube is brought into place, an AP X-ray confirms the location of the working tube on the target area (*arrow*).

approach angle, an endplate view of the caudal index-level vertebral body is obtained on anteroposterior (AP) fluoroscopy (▶ Fig. 14.2 **a**). Based on this angle, an addition of approximately 10 to 15 degrees of caudal C-arm tilt is required for the lower lumbar levels and approximately 0 to 5 degrees in the upper lumbar spine. The goal is to center the gap between the index-level spinous processes over the projection of the disk space (▶ Fig. 14.2 **a–c**). The incision is marked where the center of the disk space crosses the inferomedial edge of the rostral index-level lamina, which constitutes the *target area* of this approach (▶ Fig. 14.2 **d**). A small vertical skin incision is produced using a no. 11 blade. A trocar is then advanced with small rostrocaudal movements along the AP trajectory of the fluoroscopy until the medial aspect of the facet joint or the inferomedial margin of the lamina can be palpated. Once the trocar is in place, dilators are introduced. The dilators, in particular beveled dilators, may be used to strip muscles off the lamina and hereby facilitate the transition from palpation to visualization. Attention should be paid to keeping the dilators in solid contact with the edge of the lamina by applying gentle downward pressure. At L5/S1, the

dilators may rest on the yellow ligament. In these cases, lateral fluoroscopic images may help confirm appropriate depth (▶ Fig. 14.2 **e**). Blind penetration of the yellow ligament is not advised as it could lead to damage of neural structures. Following serial dilation, the tubular retractor is placed with the open bevel facing medially and kept in solid bone contact with the target area by applying gentle downward pressure (▶ Fig. 14.2 **f**).

14.4 Identification of Bony Landmarks

First, the inferomedial edge of the lamina (*target area*), which has been palpated with the bevel of the working tube, is visualized. To achieve this, overlying muscle and connective tissue are retraced with the bevel of the tubular retractor (used like a Cobb elevator) and resected with the bipolar cautery and micro-punches. The goal is to expose and visualize the inferomedial edge of the rostral index-level lamina (▶ Fig. 14.3 **a**). Using a diamond or side-cutting burr, lamina bone is resected along the inferomedial edge until the insertion of the yellow ligament is identified (▶ Fig. 14.3 **b**). At this point, a final AP X-ray is obtained to confirm appropriate position and level. We consider the lamina attachment of the yellow ligament the *principal anatomical landmark* for the ULBD as it guides the entire bony decompression.

14.5 Laminotomy

Utilizing a diamond burr, the central bony decompression is carried out along the insertion of the yellow ligament. For most efficient bony decompression, half of the circumference of the

diamond burr is advanced into the yellow ligament allowing the center of the burr to efficiently resect bone along the yellow ligament insertion. This technique detaches the superficial layers of the yellow ligament, which are continuously trimmed with a micro-punch or bipolar cautery to maintain visualization of the yellow ligament insertion. The bony decompression is initiated at the inferomedial aspect of the ipsilateral lamina (▶ Fig. 14.4 **a,b**). Then, the base of the spinous process is generously undercut, which is particularly important at the lower lumbar segments where the spinal canal is wide. Once the spinous process is undercut, the insertion of the yellow ligament is followed to the contralateral lamina (▶ Fig. 14.4 **c**). Utilizing a

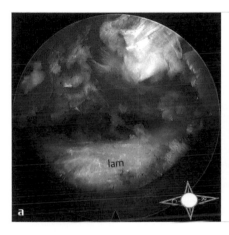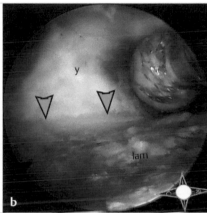

Fig. 14.3 Visualization of the *target area*. **(a)** Initially, the inferomedial edge of the lamina is exposed (lam). **(b)** Upon bony resection along the inferomedial edge of the lamina, the bony insertion (*green arrowheads*) of the yellow ligament (y) is identified (principal anatomic landmark).

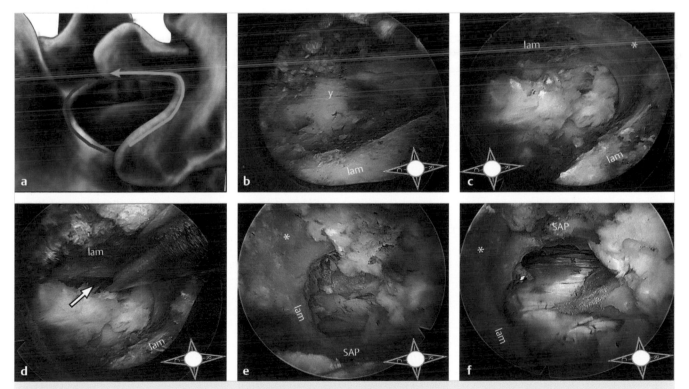

Fig. 14.4 For the laminotomy, bony decompression is carried out circumferentially along the bony insertion of the yellow ligament (*principal anatomical landmark*). **(a)** The *arrows* indicate the workflow of bony decompression. **(b)** Upon decompression of the ipsilateral lamina (lam), **(c)** the rostral spinous process (*asterisk*) is undercut and the yellow ligament attachment is followed to the contralateral lamina. **(d)** Detaching the yellow ligament with a sharp dissector exposes the ventral surface of the contralateral lamina (*arrow*). **(e)** The rostral edge of the caudal lamina is resected along the yellow ligament attachment. **(f)** Following undercutting of the caudal spinous process (*asterisk*), the rostral edge of the contralateral lamina is resected until the superior articular process (SAP) is seen (lam = lamina, y = yellow ligament).

sharp dissector, the yellow ligament is dissected off the ventral surface of the contralateral lamina (▶ Fig. 14.4 **d**). This maneuver allows us to assess the width angle of the contralateral lamina and determine the need for additional undercutting of the spinous process for appropriate access to the contralateral recess. The contralateral lamina is then undercut using the diamond burr until the facet joint is reached. At this point, resection of the caudal lamina is initiated. The rostral edge of the caudal lamina is exposed removing superficial connective tissue with the pituitary rongeurs. Once the rostral edge is visualized, bone is resected along the insertion of the yellow ligament with a diamond burr (▶ Fig. 14.4 **e**). Given the shallow attachment of the yellow ligament along the rostral edge of the lamina (see Chapter 6), the yellow ligament is typically transgressed and the epidural space is entered. The continuous irrigation utilized in full-endoscopic spine surgery retracts thecal sac and the burr can safely be utilized along the rostral edge of the caudal index-level lamina. Following undercutting of the caudal spinous process, the rostral edge of the contralateral lamina is resected until the SAP comes into view (▶ Fig. 14.4 **f**).

14.6 Flavectomy

Prior to the flavectomy, residual bony yellow ligament attachments are cauterized with the bipolar cautery to avoid cumbersome bleeding. Then, utilizing a sharp dissector or curette, the remaining yellow ligament lamina attachments are dissected off (▶ Fig. 14.5 **a,b**). Typically, the epidural space has been entered during resection of the rostral edge of the caudal

lamina. Engaging a Kerrison rongeur onto the residual yellow ligament followed by rotation and traction allows for efficient detachment of the ligamentum flavum (▶ Fig. 14.5 **c,d**). Once the ligament has been detached, a large pituitary rongeur is utilized to deliver the yellow ligament en bloc (▶ Fig. 14.5 **e,f**). Great care is taken during this maneuver to continuously inspect the dura to rule out any adhesions. Adhesions of the yellow ligament with the thecal sac may be seen in revision cases, cases with extremely severe lateral recess stenosis, large disk herniations, or synovial cysts.

14.6.1 Lateral Recess Decompression

Epidural fat, blood vessels, and yellow ligamentum within bilateral recesses are thoroughly coagulated using the bipolar cautery. The residual yellow ligament is resected with micropunches or Kerrison rongeurs. Bony decompression of the lateral recesses is carried out using Kerrison rongeurs or side-cutting burs (▶ Fig. 14.6 **a,b**). Additional undercutting of the inferior articular process may be necessary to gain access to the entire medial aspect of the SAP. In some cases, access to the medial aspect of the SAP can be facilitated by gently retracting the inferior articular process with the working sleeve. This maneuver should not be utilized in patients with osteoporosis as it may fracture the inferior articular process. Using Kerrison rongeurs or side-cutting burs, the medial aspect of the SAP is resected along the lateral margin of the neural elements (▶ Fig. 14.6 **a,b**). Utilizing this technique, a highly targeted decompression of the neural elements is accomplished

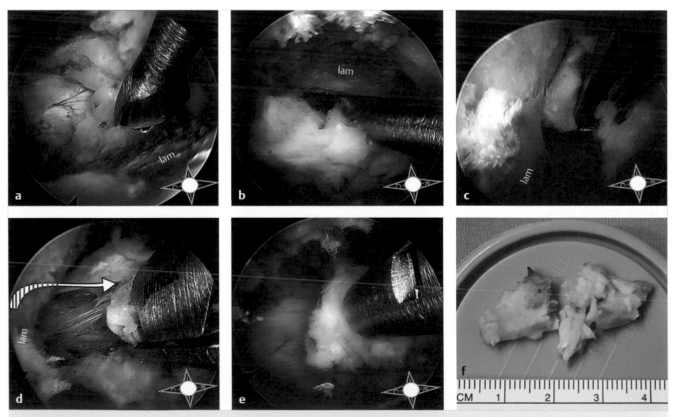

Fig. 14.5 For the flavectomy, (a) the ipsilateral and (b) contralateral lamina (lam) attachments are dissected using a sharp dissector or curette. (c) The remaining yellow ligament along the caudal lamina is detached by engaging the Kerrison rongeur, (d) followed by rotation and traction (*curved arrow*). (e) The detached yellow ligament is delivered with a pituitary rongeur en block. (f) Intraoperative yellow ligament specimen.

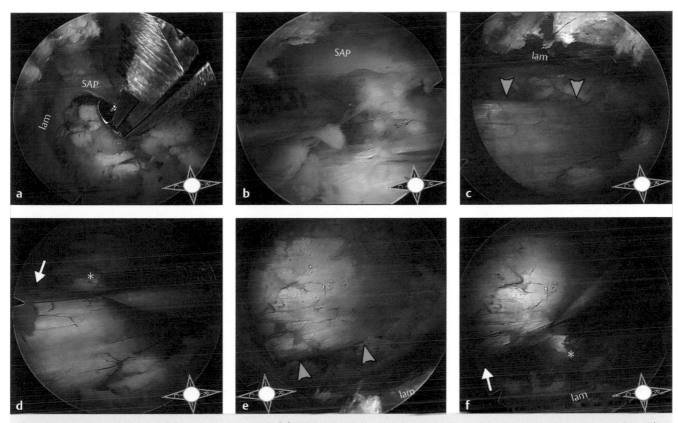

Fig. 14.6 Lateral recess decompression. The medial aspect of the superior articular process (SAP) is resected using **(a)** a Kerrison rongeur or **(b)** a side-biting burr. **(c)** Thus, the neural elements of the lateral recess (*green arrowheads*) are decompressed spanning from the tip of the SAP to the caudal pedicle. **(d)** A blunt dissector is utilized to mobilize the contralateral neural elements (*asterisk*, disk annulus). The arrow indicates the traversing nerve root. **(e)** Decompression of the ipsilateral lateral is completed, and the lateral margin of the neural elements is visualized (*green arrowheads*). **(f)** Neural elements are medialized with a blunt dissector (*asterisk*, disk annulus). The traversing nerve root (*arrow*) is decompressed spanning from the tip of the SAP to the mid-portion of the caudal pedicle. (Abbreviation: lam, lamina.)

spanning from the tip of the SAP to the mid-portion of the caudal pedicle. Using a blunt dissector, the contralateral foramen, disk, and pedicle may be palpated and then visualized. A bony decompression of the contralateral foramen can be performed if indicated (see Chapter 13).

14.6.2 Mobilization of Neural Elements

Bilateral margins of the neural elements (S1 traversing nerve root at L5/S1, L5 at L4/5, and lateral margins of the thecal sac at the lumbar levels above) are identified (▶ Fig. 14.6 **c,e**). This is easiest accomplished in the rostral aspect of the operative field (at or above the tip of the SAP). A meticulous exposure of the thecal sac with removal of epidural fat, vessels, and fascial layers greatly facilitates this step. Once visualized, a blunt dissector is used at the level of the disk space to gently medialize the lateral margin of the neural structures (▶ Fig. 14.6 **d,f**). In case of tethering, there should be a high suspicion for incomplete decompression with the traversing nerve root still trapped within an incompletely decompressed lateral recess. This is commonly encountered at L4/L5 and L5/S1. In these cases, further decompression needs to be carried out in the rostral aspect of the lateral recess until the shoulder of the traversing nerve root is identified and decompressed. Residual lateral recess stenosis is then decompressed along the

traversing nerve. Adequate decompression of neural structures should be achieved spanning from the tip of the SAP to the mid-portion of the caudal pedicle. Appearance of perineural fat tissue at the level of the caudal pedicle provides additional confirmation of a sufficient decompression.

14.7 Pearls and Pitfalls

- Case selection: Approach and bony decompression can be challenging in cases with severe spondylotic changes such as facet hypertrophy or scoliosis. If these cases are addressed with full-endoscopic technique, attention to planning the surgical corridor and unambiguous identification of the target area is critical in order to maintain a smooth workflow. Moreover, cases with scoliosis and stable spondylolisthesis require more extensive decompression to allow for sufficient decompression of neural structures during the expected physiological motion. However, once spondylolisthesis leads to symptomatic foraminal nerve root compression, reconstruction of the spinal segment via an arthrodesis procedure should be considered.
- In the upper lumbar spine, the rostrocaudal approach angle is either in line with the superior endplate of the caudal index-level or slightly more kyphotic (up to 5 degrees). At these levels, spinal stenosis is often caused by overgrowth of the

sagittally oriented facet joints. Choosing a too steep rostrocaudal approach angle may interfere with decompression of the caudal aspect of stenosis since the endoscope is deflected by caudal lamina.

- Choice of appropriate endoscope: Small-diameter (iLESSYS Pro [joimax] or interlaminar endoscope [Wolf]) versus larger-diameter endoscope (iLESSYS Delta [joimax] or Central Stenosis endoscope [Wolf]). In patients with a congenitally narrow spinal canal or in the upper lumbar spinal segments, the use of a smaller endoscope facilitates visualization, since the remaining ipsilateral facet joint may block the view obtained with the larger endoscopes. Visualization can still be obtained via rotation of the scope to allow for visualization; however, this adds difficulty to the procedure. Also, the larger endoscope makes initial docking and identification of the bony landmarks more difficult since the approach corridor may be blocked by the overgrown facet joints. However, the smaller interlaminar endoscopes are more fragile, less efficient for bone and soft-tissue resection, and more affected by hemorrhage. As a rule of thumb, we recommend using a larger Central Stenosis endoscope if the distance between the spinolaminar angle and the facet joint is equal to or larger than 1.5 cm.
- Inability to palpate target area (inferomedial edge of the lamina) with the trocar:
  - *Inaccurate radiographic targeting*: repeat AP and lateral X-rays (r/o rotation of the patient, repeat caudal AP endplate view to reset baseline).
  - *Misalignment of radiographic and surgical working corridor*: confirm alignment of the trocar with the trajectory of the AP X-ray beam.
- Inability to visualize target area with the endoscope:
  - *Suboptimal position of the tubular retractor:* repeat AP and lateral X-rays to confirm appropriate position and level.
  - *Floating up of the working tube:* make sure that the working tube is in solid contact with the target area (repeat tissue dilation and confirm the ability to palpate the target area with the bevel of the tubular retractor) or on the yellow ligament (confirm on lateral X-ray).

- *Inability to advance working tube:* The working tube might be riding on an overgrown facet joint (check on preoperative MRI). Consider using a smaller-diameter interlaminar endoscope, rotate the bevel of the working sleeve to allow for advancement, and partially resect the overgrown facet joint.
- Inability to identify yellow ligament attachment despite bony resection:
  - The bone work is done either too medial on the spinous process or too lateral within the facet joint. Confirm the trajectory of the endoscope and Obtain AP and lateral X-rays to get reoriented.
- Inability to identify dura following transgression of the yellow ligament:
  - The entry into the canal might be too lateral or in the axilla of the nerve root, in particular at L5/S1.
  - In the cases of very narrow spinal canal, in particular in upper lumbar segments, the inside of the contralateral yellow ligament can be mistaken for the thecal sac. Take a look at the mediolateral orientation of the endoscope and confirm anatomical appearance and pulsations of the thecal sac.
- Inability to define the lateral margin of the neural elements:
  - Confirm location of the working tube.
  - Widen the lateral recess decompression.
- Bone bleeding: Bleeding from small capillaries close to the articular surface may be difficult to control. Precise targeting with the bipolar cautery as well as physical pressure onto the area of bleeding helps stop bleeding. Irrigation fluid may be supplemented with epinephrine. See Chapter 8 for additional techniques to manage intraoperative bleeding.
- Contralateral recess decompression: Similar to tubular MIS decompression in cases of severe lateral recess stenosis, a very narrow lateral recess may be mistaken for the lateral aspect of the canal. Nonambiguous visualization of contralateral disk annulus and caudal pedicle helps avoid this common mistake.

15 Endoscopic Extraforaminal Lumbar Diskectomy

Christoph P. Hofstetter

15.1 Case Example

A 74-year-old man presents with a 3-month history of rapid-onset pain radiating into his left flank and left anterior thigh. The patient describes the left lower extremity pain as aching-type pain and rates the pain 7/10 in severity. He also experiences episodes of his left knee giving out, which has led to several falls. The patient had failed conservative treatments including NSAIDs (nonsteroidal anti-inflammatory drugs), physical therapy, and steroid injections. On neurological examination, his left hip flexion (4–/5) and knee extension are weak (4/5). Preoperative imaging reveals a left L3/L4 far-lateral disk herniation (▶ Fig. 15.1 **a,b**). *The procedure performed was left extraforaminal endoscopic L3/L4 diskectomy.* The patient's motor strength recovered following the procedure and his radicular pain improved.

15.2 Indications

The endoscopic extraforaminal approach utilizes a posterolateral corridor targeting the superolateral aspect of the caudal index-level pedicle. The extraforaminal endoscopic approach allows for treatment of pathology in the extraforaminal zone. Typical indications are far-lateral disk herniations or impingement of the extraforaminal nerve root by bone spurs or dislodged interbody cages. The extraforaminal approach greatly minimizes tissue manipulation when compared with traditional surgical approaches for far-lateral disk herniations. However, this approach is associated with a steep learning curve for several reasons. First, the tubular retractor floats freely in the extraforaminal space and needs to be manually held in place. Second, the extraforaminal pathology may displace the exiting nerve root inferiorly and/or medially and therefore place the nerve root at risk during docking and placement of the working tube. Finally, the extraforaminal nerve root may be difficult to visualize and identify, as it may be obscured by the pathology.

15.3 Preoperative Planning

The extraforaminal approach aims at the superolateral aspect of the caudal index-level pedicle (▶ Fig. 15.2 **a**). The distance of the skin incision from the midline is measured on preoperative axial T2-weighted MRI studies. The pathology should be accessible via a straight surgical corridor along the outside of the facet joint. As approximate guidance, the distance between the skin entry point and the midline is approximately 6 to 8 cm. The rostrocaudal approach trajectory is less steep compared to transforaminal approaches, with an inclination off approximately 5 to 10 degrees. The location of the exiting nerve root within the foramen and extraforaminal area should be carefully determined on preoperative MRI, in particular in the relation to the pathology intended to treat. Far-lateral disk herniations typically displace the nerve root rostral and lateral. However, in some cases the nerve root is displaced posteriorly and medially. In these cases, the use of a bone trephine to resect the lateral portion of the superior articular process (SAP) establishes a safe surgical corridor to bring in the endoscope.

15.4 Approach

A straight-on anteroposterior (AP) fluoroscopic image endplate view of the caudal index-level vertebral body is obtained and marked on the skin. The entry point is marked at the predetermined distance from the midline along the rostrocaudal approach trajectory. Using lateral fluoroscopy, the incision is referenced to the lateral projection of spinal column. The incision for a typical extraforaminal diskectomy is slightly dorsal to a line connecting the tips of the lumbar spinous processes. Once the entry point has been marked on the skin, a small stab incision is produced using a no. 11 blade and either an 18-G spinal needle or a Jamshidi needle is advanced toward the superolateral aspect of the caudal pedicle (*target area*) under AP and lateral fluoroscopic guidance (▶ Fig. 15.2 **a,b**). Once the appropriate target has been confirmed, a guide wire is left in place. Serial dilators are then advanced, followed by a working sleeve. The working sleeve needs to be carefully held in place and the endoscope is brought in.

15.5 Identify Bony Landmarks

First, the superolateral aspect of the caudal pedicle (*target area*) is visualized using a combination of grasping forceps, and bipolar cautery (▶ Fig. 15.3 **a**). A diamond burr may be used to resect

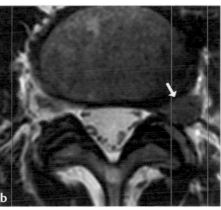

Fig. 15.1 (a) Sagittal and (b) axial T2-weighted MRI of a lumbar spine. Note the left L3/L4 far-lateral disk herniation with impingement of the exiting L3 nerve root.

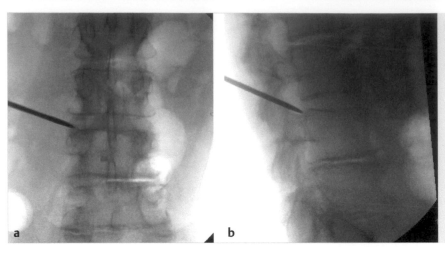

Fig. 15.2 Targeting the superolateral pedicle during a left L3/L4 extraforaminal approach shown on an **(a)** anteroposterior and **(b)** lateral fluoroscopic intraoperative images.

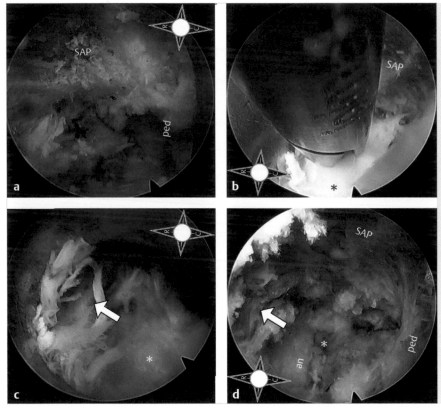

Fig. 15.3 Resection of foraminal disk herniation. **(a)** Initial view of the superolateral aspect of the caudal pedicle (ped; *target area*). **(b)** Resection of foraminal disk herniation (*asterisk*) using grasping forceps. **(c)** Following resection of the foraminal disk herniation, the perineural fat of the exiting nerve root (*arrow*) descends into the foramen (*asterisk*; residual disk herniation). **(d)** Completed foraminal decompression of the exiting nerve root (*arrow*). The annulus of the intervertebral disk (an) with an annular defect (*asterisk*) is seen (ped, pedicle, SAP, superior articular process.).

the lateral aspect of the SAP to gain access into the foramen. The Kerrison rongeur may be placed onto the rostral aspect of the caudal pedicle and appropriate location may be confirmed with fluoroscopic imaging. At this point, the superolateral aspect of the caudal pedicle, the SAP, and the posterior superior endplate of the caudal vertebral body should be identified. This concludes the approach.

15.5.1 Foraminal Decompression

First, the annulus of the intervertebral disk is identified. This is easiest accomplished by following the superior aspect of the pedicle and posterosuperior endplate of the caudal

vertebral body rostrally. Any free disk fragments may be retrieved using grasping forceps (▶ Fig. 15.3 **b**). Upon decompression, the exiting nerve root surrounded by perineal fat frequently descends into the foramen (▶ Fig. 15.3 **c**). Alternatively, the exiting nerve root can be uncovered and identified by resecting the foraminal yellow ligament (*principal anatomical landmark*) along the attachment on the SAP and pars interarticularis using a Kerrison rongeur. This maneuver is also useful in case of disk fragments rostral to the exiting nerve root. The foraminal decompression is completed once the exiting nerve root has been decompressed from the medial aspect of the caudal pedicle to the lateral aspect of the SAP (▶ Fig. 15.3 **d**).

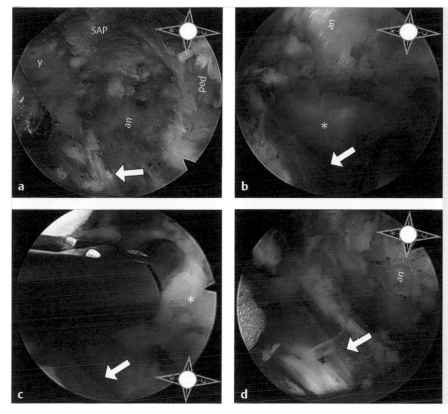

Fig. 15.4 Resection of the far-lateral disk fragment. **(a)** The exiting nerve root (*arrow*) is identified within the foramen ventral to the foraminal yellow ligament (y; *principal anatomical landmark*). The bevel of the working sleeve is rotated to lateralize the exiting nerve root in the extraforaminal area. **(b)** The disk fragment wedged underneath the exiting nerve root comes into vision (*asterisk*). **(c)** Using an up-angled cup forceps, the fragment is retrieved using a rotational movement. The exiting nerve root is decompressed in the extraforaminal area. **(d)** The annulus has been coagulated with the bipolar cautery. The arrows in **(a–d)** indicate the exiting nerve root. (Abbreviations: an, intervertebral disk annulus; ped, pedicle; SAP, superior articular process)

15.5.2 Extraforaminal Decompression

The exiting nerve root and the annulus of the intervertebral disk are followed laterally (▶ Fig. 15.4 **a**). Using the bevel of the working cannula, the extraforaminal aspect of the exiting nerve is both lateralized and gently elevated (▶ Fig. 15.4 **b**). This allows us to identify fragments that are wedged underneath the extraforaminal nerve root. If fragments are seen, then they can be gently mobilized using the bipolar cautery. Up-angled cup forceps are ideally suited to retrieve fragments from underneath the nerve. Using a rotational maneuver helps avoid any traction on the nerve root or other vital structure (perineural vasculature; ▶ Fig. 15.4 **c**). Once the fragment has been retrieved, the annular defect is explored and loose fragments are resected. The edges of the annular defect may be coagulated (▶ Fig. 15.4 **d**).

15.6 Pearls and Pitfalls

- During docking and retraction of the exiting nerve root, there is the possibility of nerve damage, which may lead to postoperative neurological deficits or paresthesias. In the cases where the nerve root is displaced posteroinferiorly by a far-lateral disk herniation, docking onto the SAP and partial resection of the lateral aspect of the SAP utilizing bone

trephines may avoid nerve root damage during placement of the working cannula.
- Typically, the exiting nerve root can be found ventral to the foraminal yellow ligament (*principal anatomical landmark*). Alternatively, it can be identified with the following strategies:
  - Resection of the foraminal yellow ligament along its attachment on the SAP and pars interarticularis will reveal the exiting nerve root.
  - Identify the traversing nerve root and follow the epidural compartment toward the exiting nerve root with the curved ball tip probe or bipolar cautery (the same maneuver that is carried out during traditional interlaminar surgery utilizing a dental tool).
  - Use intraoperative mapping. (Cathodal pulses [100 µs, 7.1/s] to elicit evoked electromyographic [EMG] responses. EMG responses can typically be detected from a threshold below 10 mA.)
  - Follow the annulus in the foramen rostrally.
- If a disk fragment is located between the rostral pedicle and the exiting nerve root, the nerve root can be crossed dorsally by resecting the yellow ligament along the foraminal attachment using a Kerrison rongeur. The insertion of the foraminal yellow ligament is followed rostrally until the rostral pedicle is reached.

16 Transforaminal Endoscopic Lumbar Diskectomy

Christoph P. Hofstetter

16.1 Case Example

A 49-year-old man presents with a 6-month history of left lower extremity pain radiating from his lower back to his buttock, lateral thigh, and lateral calf. The patient has weakness in his left gluteus medius muscle (4/5). The straight leg raise test is positive at 5 degrees in a lying position. He had failed NSAIDs (nonsteroidal anti-inflammatory drugs), physical therapy, and two steroid injections. Preoperative MRI depicts a left-sided L4/L5 disk herniation with caudal migration (▶ Fig. 16.1). *The procedure performed was a left transforaminal endoscopic L4/L5 diskectomy.* The patient's radicular pain and neurological deficit resolved postoperatively.

16.2 Indications

The transforaminal endoscopic approach utilizes a surgical corridor via the inferior aspect of the intervertebral foramen targeting the medial aspect of the foraminal annular window (Kambin's triangle). The endoscopic transforaminal approach allows for treatment of soft disk pathology located in the foramen or in the lateral recess *ventral to the traversing nerve root.* This approach allows for resection of foraminal, subarticular, and central disk herniations. Given that the traditionally trained spine surgeon is not familiar with the anatomy encountered during this approach, it has a steep learning curve. Additionally, there is the possibility of irritation/damage of the exiting nerve root, which may lead to postoperative paresthesias. Severe foraminal stenosis, facet hypertrophy, and location of the exiting nerve root within the inferior portion of the foramen increase the risk of irritation/damage of the exiting nerve root and constitute relative contraindications for this approach. In such cases, a trans-superior articular process (trans-SAP) approach should be considered. In contrast to the trans-SAP approach, the transforaminal approach targets the medial aspect of Kambin's triangle and resection of the SAP is optional. The transforaminal approach is associated with a shorter operative time and the need for less equipment compared to the trans-SAP approach (the transforaminal approach does not require bone trephines since the optional SAP resection can be performed under vision with a burr or Kerrison rongeur). The utility of the transforaminal approach may be limited at L5/S1 in particular with a steep pelvic crest. Factors that favor the transforaminal approach are large intervertebral foramen, upper lumbar segment, and a previous posterior approach.

16.3 Preoperative Planning

The transforaminal approach aims directly at the medial aspect of the foraminal annular window (*target area*, Kambin's triangle; ▶ Fig. 16.2 **a**). The distance of the skin incision from the midline is estimated on preoperative axial T2-weighted MRI studies. As approximate guidance, the distance between skin entry point and midline is approximately 12 cm at L5/S1, 10 cm at L4/L5, and 8 cm at L3/L4. When targeting pathology more medially located within the spinal canal, an entry point farther away from the midline might be selected. However, with a flat approach angle there is a higher risk of injury to the exiting nerve root. The rostrocaudal inclination depends on the location of pathology treated. For subarticular disk herniations, one of the most common indications. The inclination is determined by connecting the rostral aspect of the superior articular process and the medial aspect of the foraminal annular window. This results typically in a 15- to 25-degree rostrocaudal inclination with entrance into the intervertebral foramen adjacent to the pars interarticularis (▶ Fig. 16.2 **b**). Choosing this trajectory allows for entrance into the foramen rostral to the SAP, which avoids lateralization of the surgical corridor by the later. In the case of rostrally migrated disk, less inclination should be chosen. However, with less inclination, the transforaminal surgical corridor may be blocked by the SAP and partial resection of the SAP may be necessary. No matter what inclination is chosen, the planned trajectory should allow for inspection of the index-level disk annulus. At L5/S1, the steepness of the iliac crest needs to be considered as it makes the approach more challenging. Prior to performing a transforaminal approach, a clear understanding of the degree of facet hypertrophy as well as the precise location of the exiting nerve root is imperative. In the case of a nerve root located within the caudal aspect of the foramen, there is a high risk of impingement during placement of the trocar into the foramen and a trans-SAP or extraforaminal approach should be considered.

16.4 Approach

For general orientation, vertical lines are marked on the skin at 8, 10, and 12 cm off the midline (▶ Fig. 16.2 **a**). The intervertebral

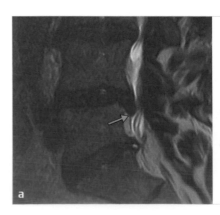
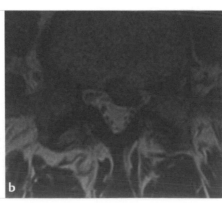

Fig. 16.1 (a) Sagittal and **(b)** axial T2-weighted MRI of the lumbar spine. Note the left L4/L5 disk herniation (*green arrow*) with impingement of the left traversing L5 nerve root.

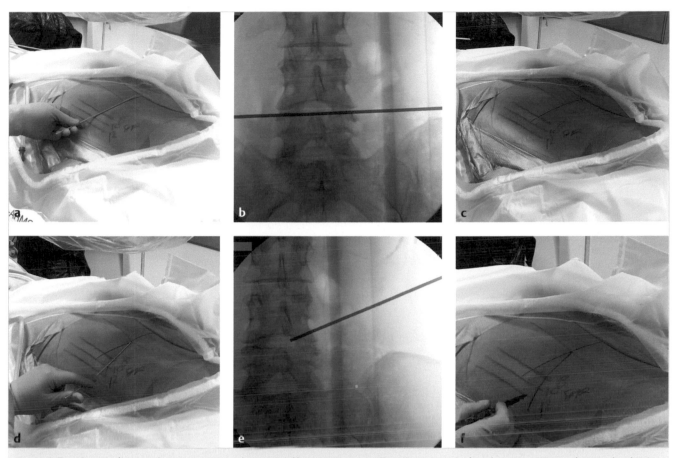

Fig. 16.2 Transforaminal approach. For orientation, three vertical lines 8, 10, 12 cm off midline are marked on the patient prior to draping. (a–c) Using a K-wire, the index disk space is determined on an anteroposterior (AP) endplate view and marked on the skin. (d–f) The rostrocaudal approach trajectory connects the rostral aspect of the superior articular process (SAP) and the medial aspect of the foraminal annular window (target area). (Continued)

disk is marked on an anteroposterior (AP) fluoroscopic endplate view of the caudal index level (▶ Fig. 16.2 **b,c**). The rostrocaudal approach trajectory, with an inclination of approximately 20 to 30 degrees, is determined by connecting the rostral aspect of the SAP and the medial aspect of the foraminal annular window (target area; ▶ Fig. 16.2 **d,e**). A tentative incision is marked where the rostrocaudal approach trajectory crosses the predetermined distance from the midline (▶ Fig. 16.2 **f**). Using lateral fluoroscopy, the incision is referenced to the lateral projection of spinal column. The incision for a standard transforaminal access should be in vicinity to a line connecting the tips of the lumbar spinous processes (▶ Fig. 16.2 **h**). Once the incision site is adjusted along the rostrocaudal approach trajectory according to the spinous process projection, either an 18-G needle or a Jamshidi needle is advanced toward the index-level foramen (▶ Fig. 16.2 **i**). The 18-G needle is typically advanced with the bevel facing ventrally and steered to the appropriate location by rotating the bevel. The Jamshidi needle is pointed toward the target area and carefully advanced. Typically, the lateral aspect of the facet joint is encountered first. The needle is then "walked" ventrally along the lateral aspect of the SAP in small steps toward the foraminal annular window (target area). Once within the foramen, the needle tip is advanced just short of the medial pedicle line (▶ Fig. 16.2 **j**). A lateral X-ray is obtained to make sure that the tip of the needle remains dorsal to the posterior vertebral line

on lateral X-ray (▶ Fig. 16.2 **k**). If the needle is within the disk at the medial pedicle line, direct visualization of the contents of the lateral recess will be hampered. In this case, either approach trajectory should be changed or a trans-SAP approach should be considered. A stab incision is produced using a no. 11 blade. A K-wire is placed, the needle withdrawn, and serial ascending size dilators are advanced to the medial pedicle line. A beveled tubular working channel is introduced with the open bevel facing the exiting nerve root and rotated to face the caudal pedicle once in the foramen. Prior to bringing in the endoscope, an X-ray is obtained to confirm the position of the tubular retractor at or slightly posterior to the posterior vertebral line (▶ Fig. 16.2 **l**).

16.5 Identify Bony Landmarks

The dilators are removed, and the endoscope is brought into the tubular retractor. Connective tissue within the lower foramen is removed using grasper forceps and the bipolar cautery. The ventrolateral surface of the SAP and the rostral surface of the caudal pedicle are exposed using the bipolar cautery and pituitary rongeur (▶ Fig. 16.3 **a**). If necessary, the opening into the lateral recess may be widened by resecting the ventral portion of the SAP using a high-speed drill or Kerrison rongeur

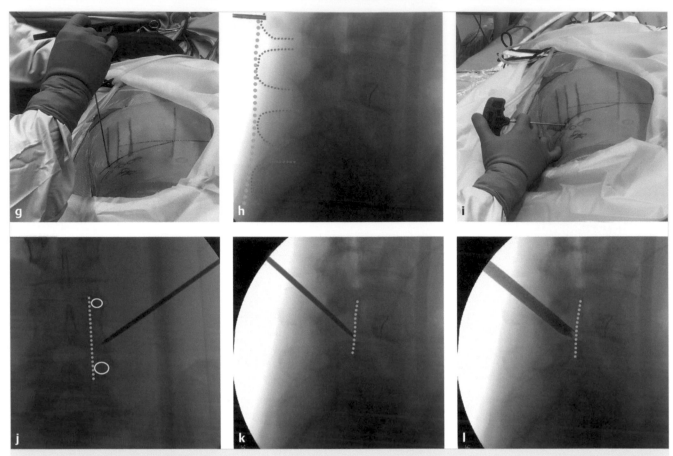

Fig. 16.2 (*Continued*) **(g)** The predetermined distance from the midline is checked on a lateral X-ray. **(h)** The skin entry point (marker in the upper left corner) should be in vicinity to a line (*green dotted line*) connecting the tips of the spinous processes (*blue dotted line*). **(i,j)** The Jamshidi needle is advanced along the rostrocaudal inclination until the facet joint is palpated. Then, the needle is moved along the lateral surface of the SAP into the foramen just short of the medial pedicle line (*green dotted line*). **(k)** A lateral X-ray is obtained to confirm that the tip of the needle remains behind the posterior vertebral line (*green dotted line*). **(l)** Following dilation and placement of the tubular retractor, another lateral X-ray confirms location within the foramen (posterior to the posterior vertebral line; *green dotted line*).

(▶ Fig. 16.3 **b**). A Kerrison rongeur may be engaged on the caudal pedicle (▶ Fig. 16.3 **c**), which allows us to both visually and radiographically confirm this *principal anatomical landmark* (▶ Fig. 16.3 **d**). This concludes the approach.

16.6 Identify the Traversing Nerve Root

In the space confined by annulus of the intervertebral disk, rostral surface of the pedicle and the ventral aspect of the SAP connective tissue is seen. The yellow ligament is easily identified since it is attached to the medioventral aspect of the SAP (▶ Fig. 16.3 **a**). Ventral to the yellow ligament, typically epidural fat becomes visible. Using the bipolar cautery, the epidural space can be entered just rostral to the pedicle, palpated (no resistance), and bluntly dissected (▶ Fig. 16.3 **e**). During the dissection, epidural fat and the traversing nerve root will come into view. Localization of the traversing nerve root is best achieved just rostral to the pedicle. In cases of severe pathology or revision surgeries, intraoperative neurophysiological map-

ping may assist with localization of the traversing nerve root. This is achieved by connecting the electrosurgical electrode (Vaporflex, Trigger-Flex) to a pulse generator and applying either monopolar or bipolar electrical stimulation. Cathodal pulses (100 μs, 2–3 Hz) are utilized to elicit evoked electromyographic (EMG) responses. EMG responses can typically be detected from a threshold of 5 mA. Once the traversing nerve root is visualized, the ventral surface of the vertebral body, posterior longitudinal ligament, and annulus of the disk may be visualized.

16.7 Resect the Disk Fragment

Using the bipolar cautery, a subarticular disk fragment is separated from the annulus (▶ Fig. 16.4 **a**). Extruded fragments may also be found intermingled with the posterior longitudinal ligament. In cases of caudally herniated disk fragments, additional resection of the superior aspect of the pedicle may be helpful. Once mobilized (▶ Fig. 16.4 **b**), the disk fragment can be retrieved using the grasping forceps. An initial rotational maneuver limits the risk of incidental damage to neural

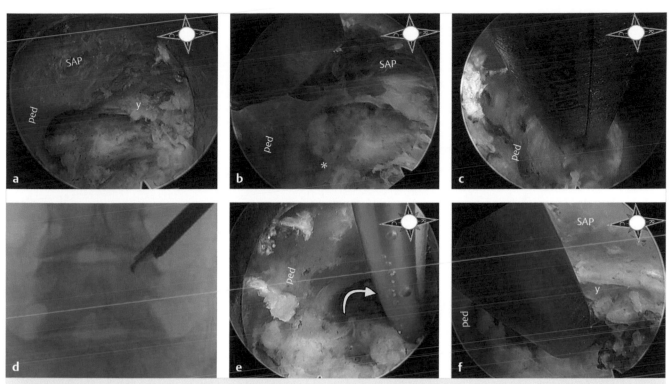

Fig. 16.3 Steps of the transforaminal approach. **(a)** The initial endoscopic view depicts the rostral surface of the caudal pedicle (ped) and the lateral aspect of the superior articulate process (SAP). **(b)** Additional resection of the ventral SAP is carried out using a cutting burr. For nonambiguous identification of the caudal index-level pedicle (*principal anatomical landmark*), **(c)** a Kerrison rongeur may be engaged over the top of the pedicle and **(d)** appropriate location is confirmed on AP X-ray. **(e)** The lateral recess in entered with the bipolar cautery just rostral to the pedicle and bluntly dissected with a rotational maneuver (*asterisk*). **(f)** Resection of the foraminal yellow ligament (y) is carried out using the Kerrison rongeur.

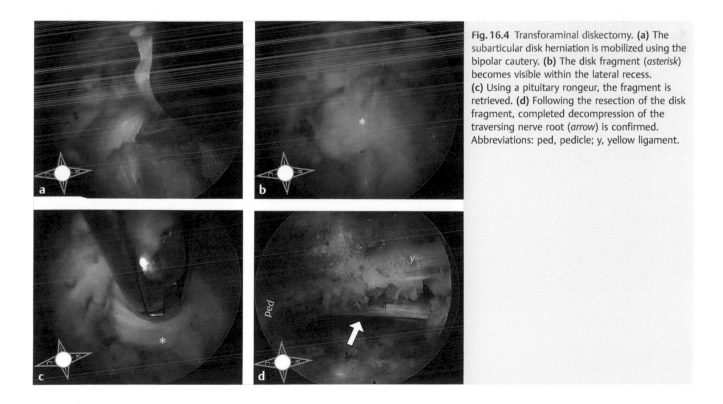

Fig. 16.4 Transforaminal diskectomy. **(a)** The subarticular disk herniation is mobilized using the bipolar cautery. **(b)** The disk fragment (*asterisk*) becomes visible within the lateral recess. **(c)** Using a pituitary rongeur, the fragment is retrieved. **(d)** Following the resection of the disk fragment, completed decompression of the traversing nerve root (*arrow*) is confirmed. Abbreviations: ped, pedicle; y, yellow ligament.

elements (▶ Fig. 16.4 **c**). Following resection of the disk herniation, the decompressed traversing nerve root is inspected (▶ Fig. 16.4 **d**).

16.8 Inspect the Annular Defect

The traversing nerve root is followed rostrally and additional yellow ligament resected as necessary. The entire rostrocaudal extent of the annulus should be inspected for annular defects. Any loose fragments should be retrieved. The edge of the remaining disk may be charred using the bipolar cautery.

16.9 Pearls and Pitfalls

- Approach: 18-G needle versus Jamshidi needle:
  - The advantage of the 18-G needle is that it may be steered by rotating the shaft. Importantly, the 18-G needle has a small diameter and should cause only minimal irritation in case of nerve contact.
  - The Jamshidi needle allows "point-and-shoot" targeting. It provides better tactile feedback. Finally, it can be advanced into the bone in case the approach needs to be converted to a trans-SAP technique.
- Approach—rostrocaudal inclination:
  - Steep rostrocaudal inclination (enter foramen adjacent to the pars interarticularis—trans-isthmus approach). This approach is ideally suited for segments with large foramen with only minimal SAP hypertrophy. It provides excellent access to downward migrated disk herniations. However, access to the rostral portion of the annulus can be limited

by deflection of the endoscope on the rostral index-level transverse process. The ideal indication for this approach is a subarticular disk herniation in a young patient.
  - Flat rostrocaudal inclination (enter the foramen lateral to the SAP). This approach is feasible in upper lumbar segments. In lower lumbar segments, entrance to the foraminal annular window may be blocked by the SAP. Thus, docking and partial resection of the SAP is necessary in order to avoid injury to the exiting nerve root. We refer to this approach as trans-SAP approach (see Chapter 17). This trajectory is ideal for central and rostrally migrated disk fragments.
- The tip of the needle is ventral to the posterior vertebral line at the medial pedicle line: At this point, do not proceed with the next steps. Most likely, the needle has been deflected ventrally by an overgrown SAP; the surgeon has the following options:
  - Increase inclination of the approach angle to enter the foramen rostral to the SAP (this is often not possible in degenerative cases with large overgrown facet joints) and collapsed disk spaces.
  - Move the skin entry more laterally (however, this maneuver increases the risk of damage to the exiting nerve root since the lateral projection of Kambin's triangle is smaller—see Chapter 7).
  - Convert to a trans-SAP approach—dock on the outside of the SAP and generate a surgical corridor through the SAP using bone trephines.
  - Perform an extraforaminal approach and resect the ventral aspect of the SAP under vision.

17 Trans-Superior Articular Process Endoscopic Lumbar Approach

Christoph P. Hofstetter

17.1 Case Example

A 74-year-old man with a past surgical history of an L4/L5 laminectomy 5 years ago presents with a left lower extremity L5 radiculopathy. The patient describes burning pain radiating from his lower back, left buttock, lateral thigh, and lateral calf. On neurological examination, his left gluteus medius (3/5) and extensor halluces longus (3/5) are found to be weak. Preoperative MRI demonstrates left L4/L5 lateral recess stenosis with impingement of the traversing L5 nerve root (▶ Fig. 17.1 **a,b**). The radicular nature of his symptoms was confirmed with an L5 diagnostic block, which gave the patient complete transient relief. *The procedure performed was left transforaminal endoscopic L4/L5 lateral recess decompression.* Postoperative CT confirmed adequate decompression of the lateral recess (▶ Fig. 17.1 **c,d**) and the patient's radicular pain and neurological deficit resolved.

17.2 Indications

The trans-superior articular process (trans-SAP) approach utilizes a posterolateral approach corridor through the SAP aiming at the lateral recess. The endoscopic trans-SAP approach allows to address bony pathology in the foramen, lateral recess, and central canal. In contrast to the transforaminal approach, it provides access to both the ventral and the dorsal aspects of the traversing nerve root. The trans-SAP allows for efficient decompression of degenerative foraminal or lateral recess stenosis. Even at L5/S1 with a steep pelvic crest, the trans-SAP is possible in most individuals. The trans-SAP approach has several advantages compared to a standard transforaminal approach. First, anchoring the Jamshidi needle in the SAP during the approach decreases the risk of aberrant foraminal bone reaming and associated risk of nerve root injury. Therefore, the trans-SAP approach may be a safer procedure during the initial period of the learning curve. Second, the trans-SAP approach can be safely performed even in cases of severely overgrown facet joints or exiting nerve roots located within the inferior portion of the foramen. Third, a wider approach corridor via the SAP decreases the rate of irritation of the exiting nerve root with possibly fewer postoperative paresthesias compared to the transforaminal approaches. Fourth, direct visualization of lateral recess including the ventral and dorsal aspects of the

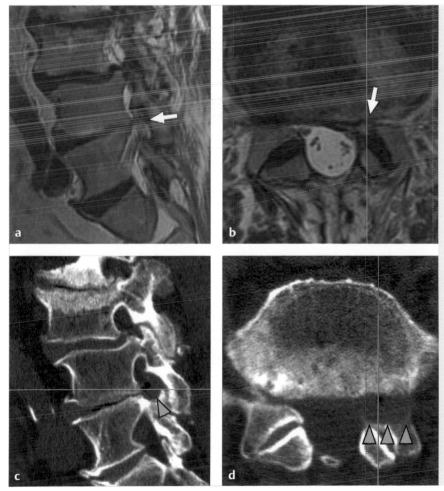

Fig. 17.1 Preoperative (a) sagittal and (b) axial T2-weighted MRI depicts left L4/L5 lateral recess stenosis with impingement of the traversing L5 nerve root (*arrows*). Postoperative (c) sagittal and (d) axial CT scans confirm resection of the superior articular process and successful decompression of the lateral recess (*green arrowheads*).

traversing nerve root allows for thorough decompression of the lateral recess. Disadvantages of this approach include a steep learning curve since the approach angle and intraoperative visualization are novel to traditionally trained spine surgeons. Moreover, additional bone work during the trans-SAP approach increases the operative time and requirement for equipment (bone trephines and burrs for partial SAP resection). Factors that favor the trans-SAP approach include the following: lower lumbar segment, foraminal stenosis, overgrown facet joints, location of the exiting nerve root in the inferior aspect of the foramen, lateral recess pathology, combined foraminal and lateral recess pathology, as well as a previous posterior approach.

17.3 Preoperative Planning

The trans-SAP approach aims directly at the lateral recess with the approach corridor traversing the SAP (▶ Fig. 17.2). The location of the skin incision is carefully planned on preoperative MRI. As approximate guidance, the distance between skin entry point and midline is approximately 12 cm at L5/S1, 10 cm at L4/L5, and 8 cm at L3/L4. Utilizing axial T2-weighted MRI, the distance of skin entry point to the midline is determined and the amount of SAP removal is estimated (▶ Fig. 17.2). For safety, the skin entry point should be referenced to the lateral projection of spinous process and/or facet joints in an axial MRI. Typically, the skin entry point is slightly ventral to the lateral projection of the tip of the spinous process but dorsal to the facet joints (▶ Fig. 17.2). The rostrocaudal approach angle depends on the type and location of pathology treated. Foraminal pathology, lateral recess stenosis, nonmigrated disk herniations, and endoscopic interbody fusions are best carried out with a rostrocaudal angle in line or slightly steeper than the disk space (5 degrees). Caudal disk herniations can be approached with a steeper rostrocaudal trajectory. At L5/S1, the steepness of the

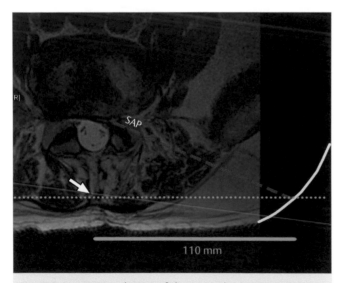

Fig. 17.2 Preoperative planning of the approach trajectory on an axial T2-weighted MRI. The approach trajectory is marked with the interrupted *red dotted line*. It aims onto the lateral recess via the superior articular process (SAP; *target area*). The skin incision is planned where the lateral projection of the tip of the spinous process (*arrow*) intersects with the skin surface (*white line*). The incision in this case is approximately 110 mm lateral to the midline (*green line*).

iliac crest needs to be considered as it makes the approach more difficult. Prior to a trans-SAP approach, a clear understanding of the degree of facet hypertrophy as well as the precise location of the exiting nerve root is imperative.

17.4 Approach

An anteroposterior (AP) fluoroscopic endplate view of the caudal vertebral body of the index level is obtained (▶ Fig. 17.3 **a**). Then, the skin is marked along a radiopaque marker aiming toward the lateral recess with a slight rostrocaudal inclination. A tentative skin incision is marked where the predetermined distance from the midline crosses this line. The skin incision is referenced to the lateral projection of the tips of the lumbar spinous processes on a lateral X-ray (▶ Fig. 17.3 **b**). Typically, the entry point for a trans-SAP approach is slightly ventral to the tips of the lumbar spinous processes. Lateral X-ray verification of the entry point in relation to the bony anatomy is particularly important in slim patients with the flank curving sharply ventrally off-midline. Thus, lateral X-ray verification prevents the selection of an entry point ventral to posterior the vertebral line that would risk injury to retroperitoneal structures. A small stab incision is produced using a no. 11 blade and a Jamshidi needle is advanced toward the SAP of the facet joint under AP fluoroscopic guidance. Once the Jamshidi needle docks on the facet joint, an AP X-ray is obtained to adjust the rostrocaudal approach trajectory (▶ Fig. 17.3 **c**). Then, a lateral X-ray is taken and the dorsoventral docking point of the Jamshidi needle is adjusted (▶ Fig. 17.3 **d**). Ideally, the Jamshidi needle is anchored in the mid-portion of the SAP (*target area*) at the level of the disk space. Using a mallet, the Jamshidi needle is advanced and ventral "progression" of the Jamshidi needle within the SAP should be observed on lateral fluoroscopic imaging. The Jamshidi needle is advanced to the medial pedicle line (▶ Fig. 17.3 **e**). Once in place, a lateral X-ray needs to be obtained to make sure that the tip of the Jamshidi needle is dorsal to the posterior vertebral line (▶ Fig. 17.3 **f**). The goal is to have the Jamshidi needle point toward the lateral recess (a view through Jamshidi needle would reveal the traversing nerve root in the center). Ascending size dilators and bone trephines (TESSYS Access Kit, joimax) are then used to partially resect the SAP and to create the trans-SAP working corridor. During the reaming, advancement of the reamers is monitored on AP X-rays. Do not advance beyond the medial pedicle line in the lower lumbar segments and beyond the middle of the pedicle in the upper lumbar segments as reamers could damage the traversing nerve root (▶ Fig. 17.3 **g**; see Chapter 25). Once the reaming has been completed, a final lateral X-ray confirms that the tip of the largest diameter reamer is dorsal of the posterior vertebral line (▶ Fig. 17.3 **h**). Once completed, a beveled tubular working channel is introduced with the open bevel facing the exiting nerve root and then rotated to face the caudal pedicle once in place.

17.5 Identify Bony Landmarks

The dilators are removed, and the endoscope is brought into the tubular working channel. Bone and connective tissue debride produced by the bone trephines are removed using grasper forceps. The ventrolateral surface of the SAP (*target area*) and

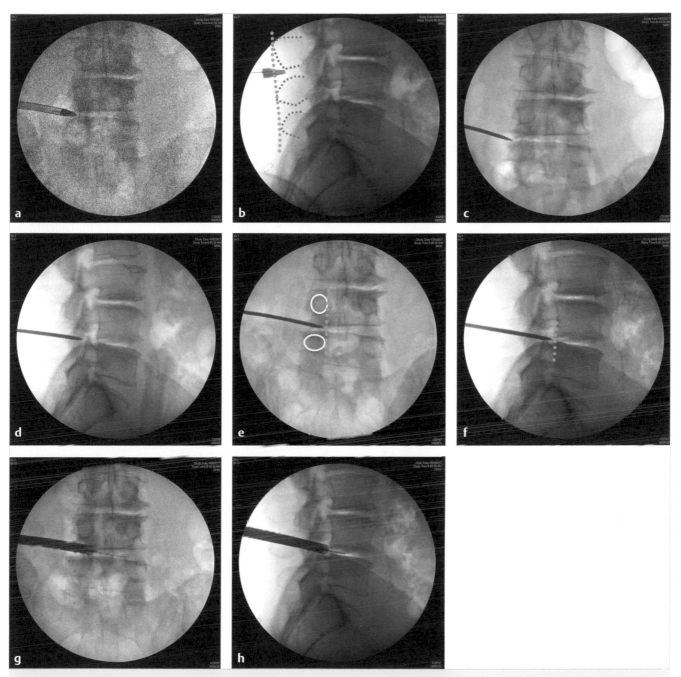

Fig. 17.3 Trans-superior articular process (trans-SAP) targeting and reaming steps as monitored with fluoroscopy. First, an endplate view of the caudal segment is obtained. **(a)** The skin is marked along the radiopaque marker with a slight rostrocaudal inclination. The intersection between this line and the predetermined distance from the midline is marked as the incision. **(b)** The skin entry point should be slightly ventral to a line (*green dotted line*) drawn through the tip of the spinous processes (*blue dotted line*) on a lateral X-ray. **(c)** A Jamshidi needle is advanced via the skin incision until the lateral aspect of the SAP (*target area*) is palpated. **(d)** The dorsoventral location of the docking point is adjusted on a lateral X-ray. **(e)** The Jamshidi needle is advanced toward the medial pedicle line (*green dotted line*) and **(f)** a lateral X-ray confirms that the tip of the Jamshidi needle remains dorsal to the posterior vertebral line (*green dotted line*). **(g)** Serial dilators and bone trephines are advanced under anteroposterior fluoroscopic guidance. **(h)** Appropriate position of the tip of the tubular retractors is verified one more time on a lateral X-ray.

the superior aspect of the caudal pedicle that have been partially resected with the bone trephines are visualized (▶ Fig. 17.4 **a**). A curved drill such as the Deflectable Shrill (joimax) or Tip-Control Articulating Burr System (Wolf) may be used to resect the ventral aspect of the SAP along the attachment of the yellow ligament (▶ Fig. 17.4 **b**). Bone resection is carried out using a circular motion from the rostral aspect of the pedicle toward

the SAP. Once the resection is completed, the pedicle and the remaining SAP create a bony "arch," which opens into the lateral recess. Careful inspection of the bony structure typically reveals the increased cortical thickness along the arch at the transition from SAP to the pedicle (▶ Fig. 17.4 **a**). For unmistakable identification of the caudal pedicle, a Kerrison rongeur may be placed onto the rostral aspect of the pedicle (▶ Fig. 17.4 **c**)

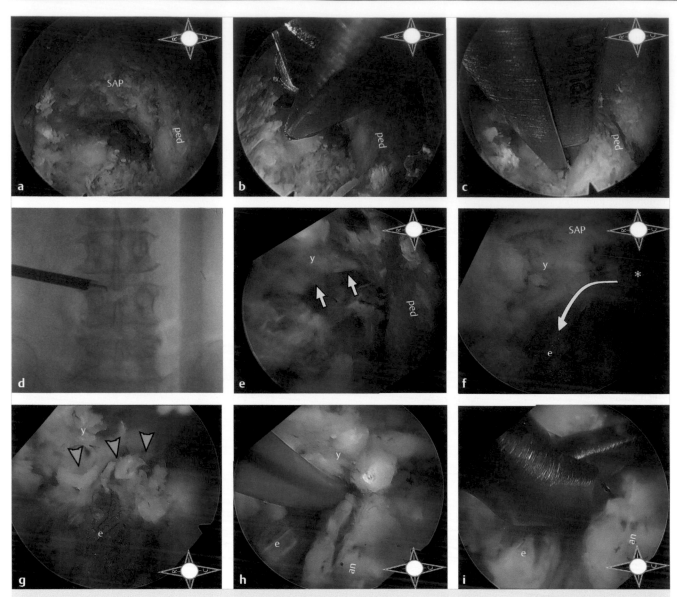

Fig. 17.4 Foraminal decompression. **(a)** Initial view of the rostral aspect of the pedicle (ped) and ventrolateral surface of the superior articular process (SAP). **(b)** Using an articulating burr, the rostral portion of the SAP is resected. Once the pedicle–SAP arch becomes visible, **(c)** a Kerrison rongeur is placed onto the rostral surface of the pedicle and **(d)** an AP X-ray is obtained for unambiguous identification of this *principal anatomical landmark*. **(e)** The yellow ligament attached to the medioventral surface of the SAP is seen (y). The epidural space is found ventral to the edge of the yellow ligament *(arrows)*. **(f)** The yellow ligament is followed rostrally until the perineural fat of the exiting nerve root (e) is seen. The epidural space of traversing nerve root (*asterisk*) is bluntly dissected with the curved bipolar and followed to the compartment of the exiting nerve root in the foramen (*curved arrow*). **(g)** The exiting nerve root (e) is decompressed by resecting foraminal yellow ligament (y) and undercutting the pars interarticularis (*green arrowheads*). **(h)** The exiting nerve root (e) is dissected off the foraminal disk annulus (an). **(i)** The bulging foraminal annulus (an) is resected using a micro-punch.

and an AP X-ray is obtained (▶ Fig. 17.4 **d**). The caudal index-level pedicle constitutes the *principal anatomical landmark* for the trans-SAP approach.

17.5.1 Decompression of the Intervertebral Foramen

The yellow ligament, which is attached to the ventromedial surface of the SAP and forms the posterior confinement of the lateral recess, is identified (▶ Fig. 17.4 **e**). Using a Kerrison rongeur, the yellow ligament may be resected along the edge of the

SAP. This exposes the epidural space, filled with fat tissue. Using the bipolar probe, the epidural space may be entered just rostral to the caudal index-level pedicle. Typically, there is little to no resistance to blunt dissection of the epidural space. Epidural fat may be carefully resected using grasping forceps and bipolar cautery until the traversing nerve root comes into view. If visualization of the nerve root is hampered by aberrant anatomy, pathology, or scar tissue, intraoperative neurophysiological mapping may assist with localization of the traversing nerve root. This is achieved by connecting the electrosurgical electrode (Vaporflex, Trigger-Flex) to a pulse generator and applying either monopolar or bipolar electrical stimulation. Cathodal pulses (100 µs; 2–3 Hz) are utilized to elicit evoked electromyographic (EMG) responses. EMG responses can typically be detected from a threshold below 10 mA. For exposure of the exiting nerve root, the ventral edge of the yellow ligament (*arrows* in ▶ Fig. 17.4 **e**) is followed rostrally into the rostral portion of the foramen. Resection of the yellow ligament often exposes the perineural fat of the exiting nerve root (▶ Fig. 17.4 **f**). If the compartment of the exiting nerve root does not readily come into view, it can be identified by following the epidural space of the lateral recess into the foraminal compartment of the exiting nerve root utilizing the curved bipolar cautery (▶ Fig. 17.4 **f**). Once the exiting nerve root has been identified, compressing foraminal yellow ligament dorsal to the nerve root can be resected along its insertion on the pars interarticularis using the Kerrison rongeur or micro-punches (▶ Fig. 17.4 **g**). If the nerve root is compressed by a foraminal disk bulge, the nerve root is dissected off the annulus using the bipolar cautery (▶ Fig. 17.4 **h**). The bulging disk may then be resected using straight or up-angled micro-punches (▶ Fig. 17.4 **i**). The extent of the foraminal soft tissue and bony decompression in relation to the exiting nerve root is inspected and completed as necessary. Upon sufficient decompression, the exiting nerve root commonly expands into lower portions of the foramen. During direct decompression of the exiting nerve root, great care should be taken to avoid extensive pressure onto the dorsal root ganglion which could cause postoperative paresthesias. Moreover, injury

of the perineural arterial vessels should be avoided since bleeding can be difficult to control.

17.5.2 Decompression of the Lateral Recess

The entry to the lateral recess is confined by annulus of the intervertebral disk, rostral surface of the pedicle, and the ventral aspect of the SAP (▶ Fig. 17.5 **a**). Typically, yellow ligament, connective tissue, or fat tissue are encountered in this region. The yellow ligament is easily identified given its attachment to the medioventral aspect of the SAP forming the dorsal boundary of the lateral recess. Ventral to the yellow ligament, epidural fat of the lateral recess may be visible (▶ Fig. 17.5 **a**). Using the bipolar cautery, the epidural space can be entered just rostral to the caudal pedicle. The epidural space may be palpated (minimal resistance) and bluntly dissected. During the dissection, the traversing nerve root typically comes into vision (▶ Fig. 17.5 **b**). In cases of aberrant anatomy, pathology (such as large disk herniations), or scar tissue, intraoperative neurophysiological mapping may be helpful to safely identify the traversing nerve root. Dorsal decompression of the traversing nerve root is accomplished by resecting the ventral aspect of the SAP. Resection of the SAP is carried out along the attachment of the yellow ligament utilizing an articulating burr (▶ Fig. 17.5 **c**). The

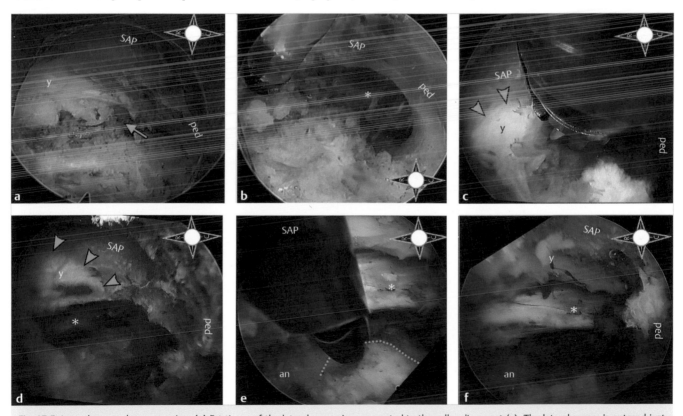

Fig. 17.5 Lateral recess decompression. **(a)** Fat tissue of the lateral recess is seen ventral to the yellow ligament (y). The lateral recess is entered just rostral to the caudal index-level pedicle (ped; *green arrow*). **(b)** Utilizing the bipolar cautery, epidural fat is dissected off bluntly from the traversing nerve root (*asterisk*). **(c)** Dorsal decompression of the lateral recess is accomplished using an articulating drill, resecting superior articular process (SAP) along the insertion of the yellow ligament (*green arrowheads*). **(d)** Once the bony dorsal decompression is completed, the yellow ligament is seen dorsal to traversing nerve root (*asterisk*). **(e)** Ventral decompression of the lateral recess is accomplished by resecting a prominent posterosuperior marginal osteophyte of the caudal index level (*green dotted line*) using a side-biting burr (an, annulus of the intervertebral disk). **(f)** Complete dorsal and ventral decompression of the traversing nerve root has been achieved.

yellow ligament that protects the traversing nerve root during the use of the burr may be resected with a Kerrison rongeur or up-angled micro-punch once the bony decompression is complete (▶ Fig. 17.5 **d**). Pathology ventral to the nerve root such as bulging disks or marginal osteophytes can also be addressed. Marginal osteophytes originating from the posterior index-level endplates can be resected using either protected side-biting burrs or diamond burrs (▶ Fig. 17.5 **e**). Upon successful lateral recess decompression, the traversing nerve root should be decompressed dorsally and ventrally spanning from the rostral aspect of the pedicle to the tip of the SAP (▶ Fig. 17.5 **f**).

17.6 Pearls and Pitfalls

- Docking the Jamshidi needle on the lateral aspect of the SAP: If the tip of the needle is docked on the dorsal aspect of the SAP, the bone reamers may follow the path of least resistance and enter the facet joint. If the tip is too ventral, the needle will slip off the SAP and reaming will be insufficient. Moreover, nonanchored foraminal reaming may increase the risk of nerve root injury.
- During the approach, the Jamshidi needle is advanced to the medial pedicle line (▶ Fig. 17.3 **e**) and a lateral X-ray shows that the tip of the needle is ventral to the posterior vertebral line: Placement of the tubular retractor ventral to the posterior vertebral line will prevent access to the rostral part of the caudal pedicle (*principal anatomical landmark* for this approach) and will hamper direct visualization of the lateral recess. In this case, we recommend revising the docking with the Jamshidi needle on the lateral aspect of the SAP in a more dorsal location.
- The caudal pedicle has been identified, but the exiting nerve root is difficult to visualize. The following strategies facilitate the visualization of the exiting nerve root:
  - Resection of the foraminal yellow ligament along its attachment on the SAP and pars interarticularis will reveal the exiting nerve root.
  - Identify the traversing nerve root and follow the epidural compartment toward the exiting nerve root with the curved ball tip probe or bipolar cautery. (The same maneuver that is carried out during traditional interlaminar surgery utilizing a dental tool.)
  - Use intraoperative mapping. (Cathodal pulses [100 µs, 7.1/s] to elicit evoked EMG responses. EMG responses can typically be detected from a threshold below 10 mA.)
  - Follow the annulus in the foramen rostrally.
- Elevate foraminal yellow ligament with the articulating jaw of a pituitary rongeur to visualize the exiting nerve root.
- The caudal pedicle has been identified, but the traversing nerve root is difficult to visualize (typical for revision lateral recess decompression or large disk herniations):
  - Resect some bone of the rostral aspect of the pedicle. The traversing nerve root is typically found just medial to the pedicle.
  - Resect the yellow ligament attached to the SAP. The epidural space is ventral to the yellow ligament.
  - Use neurophysiological mapping to identify the traversing nerve root.

18 Transforaminal Endoscopic Lumbar Interbody Fusion

Michael Y. Wang

18.1 Indications

Interbody fusion is a highly effective technique for treating a variety of disorders of the lumbar spine. Because the technique involves disk removal, cage placement, interbody height restoration, and intersegmental fusion, numerous pathologies can be treated, including segmental instability, mild deformity, and vertical foraminal stenosis. Open interbody fusion is also commonly combined with direct decompression of the neural elements in the central canal or foramen. However, we do not routinely include a unilateral laminotomy for bilateral decompression with a transforaminal endoscopic lumbar interbody fusion as this would require the use of a different endoscope (interlaminar) and a different approach trajectory and would significantly increase the operative time. Spine surgeons have become very familiar with the anatomy of the transforaminal lumbar interbody approach as it is the surgical corridor used for transforaminal lumbar interbody fusion, posterior lumbar interbody fusion, or transpedicular corpectomies. However, certain modifications are necessary when using the endoscopic approach. Most critically, since the access is through Kambin's triangle, care must be taken to avoid injury to the exiting nerve root. In addition, because the facet removal is incomplete, the use of expandable interbody is generally necessary.

18.2 Approach and Access

The operating room setup typically involves a single fluoroscopic machine. Biplanar fluoroscopy can assist with orientation for the surgeon, but becomes cumbersome in all but the largest operating rooms. An anteroposterior (AP) endplate view of the caudal index-level vertebral body is obtained showing the endplate as a single line on fluoroscopy, and the spinous process precisely centered (▶ Fig. 18.1 **a**). For transforaminal endoscopic lumbar interbody fusion, the approach corridor is typically in the plane of the disk in order to reach the contralateral side as well as to place the cage appropriately (▶ Fig. 18.1 **b**). The skin incision is planned approximately 8 to 12 cm off-midline along the projection of the index-level disk space. The distance to the midline is influenced by several factors including the size of the patient, size of the facet joint, and the spinal

segment treated. A 1-cm transverse skin incision using a no. 11 blade is made and an 18-G needle is advanced into Kambin's triangle (*target area*; see Chapter 16). In cases of overgrown facet joints or a small foramen, a trans-superior articular process (trans-SAP) technique may be utilized to gain safe access to the foraminal annular window (see Chapter 17). Advancing successive dilators over the needle/guidewire system allows for a final port of 7 to 8 mm in diameter. Ports of larger diameter can also be used, but it increases the risk of impingement of the dorsal root ganglion of the exiting nerve root.

18.3 Diskectomy and Endplate Preparation

If necessary, direct decompression of the ipsilateral foramen and/or recess may be carried out as described in Chapter 18. It should be added that in the setting of an interbody fusion, the patient benefits from the effects of indirect decompression. Restoring interbody disk space height can achieve both central canal decompression and bilateral neuroforaminal decompression in select cases. This beneficial effect is particularly seen in patients with spondylolisthesis. Because one of the major goals of the procedure is achieving a successful arthrodesis, the preparation of the graft recipient site is critical. Even in the best of hands, the extent of intervertebral disk resection in open transforaminal lumbar interbody fusions will be less than 60%. Clearly performing a diskectomy through a 7- to 9-mm port constitutes a major limitation and requires meticulous attention to detail. This is a result not only of the small working channel, but also of the inability to approach the disk at multiple angles and trajectories. To assist with adequate disk clearance, the endoscopic surgeon will need to utilize specialized tools. We typically restore the disk height using serial dilators. Then a blunt drill is utilized to deliver central disk material (▶ Fig. 18.2 **a**). Off-axis disk material is delivered utilizing pituitary rongeurs and automated brushes (▶ Fig. 18.2 **b**). The endplate preparation can be inspected directly using the endoscope (▶ Fig. 18.2 **c**). The allover extent of disk removal can also be radiographically confirmed by filling a balloon with radiopaque dye within the diskectomy site to confirm not only

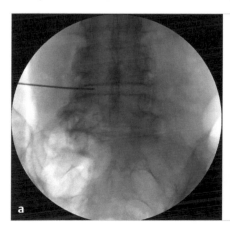
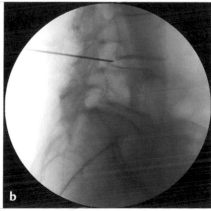

Fig. 18.1 Intraoperative approach planning for transforaminal endoscopic lumbar interbody fusion. **(a)** Anteroposterior (AP) and **(b)** lateral fluoroscopic images showing the proper placement of the spinal needle in "true" AP and lateral views to access Kambin's triangle. Note that the needle tip is localized at the medial pedicle line while remaining behind the posterior vertebral line.

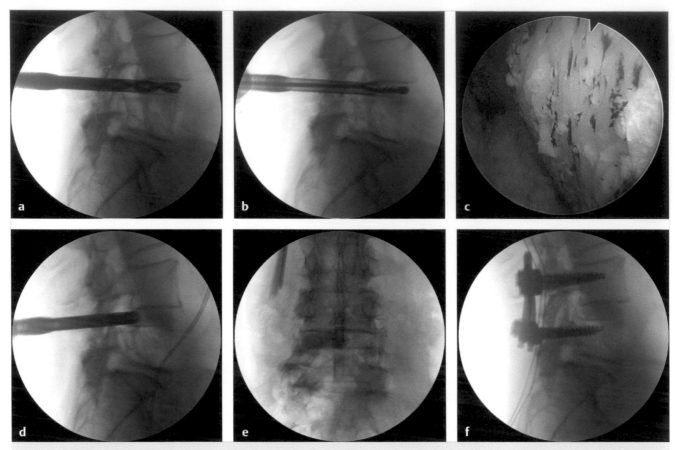

Fig. 18.2 Disk removal in preparation for interbody fusion using **(a)** a large drill to provide initial access and **(b)** automated steel brushes to prepare the endplate bone. **(c)** The prepared endplate can be inspected directly using the endoscope. The extent of disk removal can be checked using a balloon filled with contrast dye on **(d)** anteroposterior (AP) and **(e)** lateral X-ray prior to **(f)** final cage placement.

the extent of disk removal but also the potential areas/locations that need to be addressed (▶ Fig. 18.2 **d,e**).

18.3.1 Interbody Cage Placement and Osteobiologics

After preparation of the disk space, the surgeon can insert osteobiologics and an intervertebral cage device. Various osteobiologics can be used, but given the need for successful arthrodesis in order to maintain long-term results, the surgeon will need to pick carefully. Numerous cage devices are also available, and given the small size of the access port, expandable options are usually best (▶ Fig. 18.3). The use of expandable cages can also enhance interbody height restoration and allow for the most efficient indirect decompression (▶ Fig. 18.4 **a,b**).

18.3.2 Percutaneous Screw Fixation and Spondylolisthesis Correction

Numerous methods for screw placement are available, including the following:
- AP-only targeting.
- Biplanar fluoroscopy.
- Owls eye en face approach for cannulation.
- Image guidance.

In general, percutaneous screw placement is followed by submuscular rod passage to create a screw–rod construct to enhance stabilization and facilitate arthrodesis. Various maneuvers can be used to correct spondylolisthesis if the cage placement and expansion have not been sufficient for this. Generally, just connecting the screws to the rod will provide some degree of correction. In addition, an extension maneuver will mobilize the cranial segment posteriorly, reducing the slippage by at least one Meyerding grade (▶ Fig. 18.4 **c,d**).

18.3.3 Postoperative Care

As with any spinal fusion procedure, the patient should be given perioperative antibiotics and taught how to mobilize with a physical therapist. The typical hospital stay will be overnight, but there is great potential for this procedure to be performed in an outpatient ambulatory surgery center. We recommend external bracing when out of bed for a total of 12 weeks after surgery. Standard radiographic imaging is obtained every 3 months until a solid arthrodesis is confirmed.

18.4 Pearls and Pitfalls

- Skin incision: The entry site for access to the intervertebral disk must be located at the correct location to minimize nerve root injury, yet allow access to the midline of the

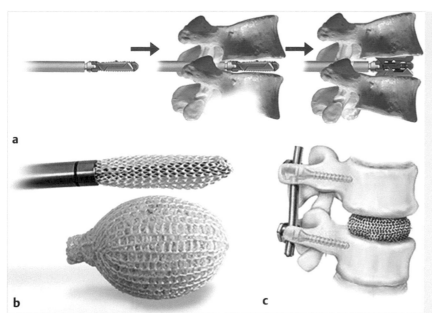

Fig. 18.3 Examples of expandable interbody cages. **(a)** A mechanical micro-machined expandable titanium cage that elevates in situ. **(b,c)** A fillable cage is internally packed with allograft growing in three dimensions and placed into the disk space.

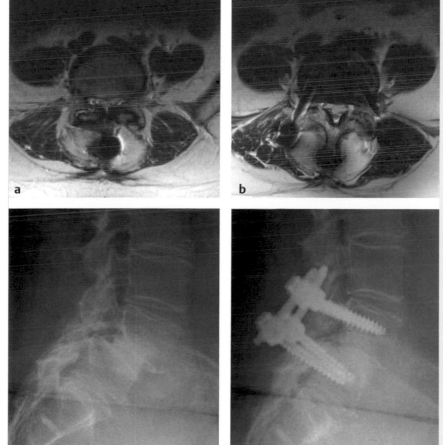

Fig. 18.4 Examples of indirect decompression and reduction of deformity. **(a)** Preoperative and **(b)** postoperative T2-weighted axial MRI scans showing the effects of indirect decompression upon interbody height restoration. **(c,d)** A grade 2 L4/L5 spondylolisthesis is corrected using placement of an expandable cage and rod–screw maneuvers.

intervertebral disk. The greater the distance of the incision to the midline, the farther the surgeon can reach to the contralateral side of the disk space. However, the more horizontal the approach angle, the higher the risk of impinging upon the dorsal root ganglion of the exiting nerve root. Contacting the facet joint bone during placement of the spinal needle will allow the surgeon to "walk" the needle tip ventrally along the lateral aspect of the SAP in small steps to be as close to the facet joint as possible. This maneuver maximizes the distance to the exiting nerve root. In spinal segments with severely hypertrophic facet joints, bone trephines may be utilized to resect the lateral aspect of the SAP, allowing access into the wider medial portion of Kambin's triangle.

- Docking point: The needle tip should enter the annulus fibrosus of the disk as close to the lateral aspect of the SAP as possible and as caudally as possible to minimize nerve injuries.
- Nerve root monitoring: Surgeons can choose to use electrophysiologic monitoring via the needle tip or to perform the surgery under analgo-sedation to detect any nerve root impingement. This is important even in the setting of perfect radiographic localization, as conjoined or abnormal nerve root anatomy may put these structures in jeopardy.
- Interbody graft movement and displacement can be the result of inadequate disk and cartilaginous endplate removal.
- Direct endoscopic inspection of the vertebral body endplates assists in confirming adequate disk removal and endplate preparation.

- The cage can generally only be placed in locations where disk removal is adequate. Thus, if a cage must cross the midline, the disk cartilage in the midline must be cleared at a minimum.
- The removal of the entire disk using only endoscopic equipment can be laborious and time-consuming. Thus, clearing enough of a path so that the removal can be centered on a narrow cleared area in the right orientation allows for use of automated disk removal tools to be effective under fluoroscopic guidance instead of direct visualization. Since most disk removal tracts will simply remove cartilage radially away from the center of the initial path, the creation of the proper initial tract (under direct visualization) is very helpful for proper cage placement.
- Cage placement can be central or asymmetric depending on the clinical and radiographic needs of the surgeon.
- Powerful expandable cages carry the risk of endplate violation, particularly in patients with osteoporosis. Inadvertent endplate violations may result in cage subsidence and loss of indirect decompression.
- The use of rhBMP-2 (recombinant human bone morphogenetic protein-2) can be a powerful adjunct to enhance fusion. However, careful attention to dosing is needed to prevent osteolysis and heterotopic bone formation. Generally, the osteobiologic needs to be placed away from the neural elements, and doses of less than 2.1 mg per spinal segment should be used.

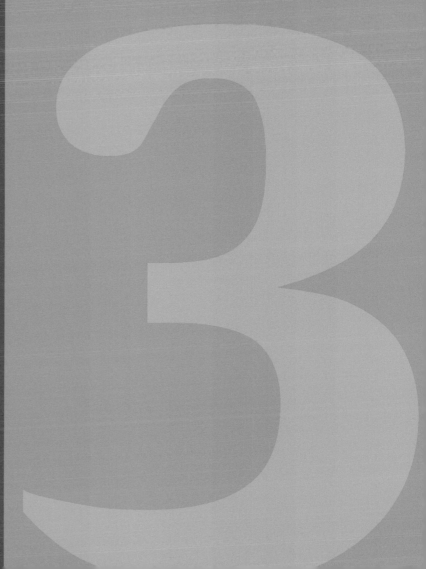

Part 3

Thoracic

19 Transforaminal Endoscopic Thoracic Diskectomy

Christoph P. Hofstetter

19.1 Case Example

A 69-year-old woman with a past medical history of Guillain–Barré syndrome, and viral meningitis as well as a surgical history of a T12/L1 instrumented fusion and attempted decompression of a large central disk herniation complicated by a cerebrospinal fluid (CSF) leak 1 year ago presents with progressive myelopathy. The patient complains about bilateral lower extremity (LE) pain that she rates as 8/10. She describes constant bilateral LE muscle cramps, has difficulties walking, and has progressive bladder urgency. On neurological examination, the patient has intact LE motor strength except for weakness in her left knee extension (4 + /5). The patient has a left positive Babinski sign. The preoperative MRI demonstrates a large disk herniation eccentric to the left at T12/L1 with impingement of the spinal cord (▶ Fig. 19.1 **a,b**). *The procedure performed was left transforaminal endoscopic T12/L1 diskectomy.* The patient tolerated the procedure well and was discharged home on the first postoperative day. Postoperative MRI confirmed resection of the disk protrusion and adequate decompression of the spinal cord (▶ Fig. 19.1 **c,d**). More than 1 year after the surgery, the patient's LE pain has greatly improved, and she rates the pain as 1/10. Her muscle cramps have resolved and she is able to walk for up to 5 hours. She still has difficulties walking downstairs but is working actively with physical therapy to improve her balance.

19.2 Indications

Thoracic disk herniations are traditionally approached via either a transpedicular or an anterior transthoracic approach. The endoscopic transforaminal approach greatly minimizes the invasiveness of this procedure by providing access to the spinal canal ventral to the spinal cord without the need for facet joint/pedicle removal or access of the thoracic cavity. Considering the anatomy of thoracic spine and adjoining ribs, the approach angle is limited; however, optimization of the skin incision and performing a foraminoplasty allows for access to the entire extent of the spinal canal ventral to the spinal cord. Depending on body habitus, this approach may be challenging in the upper thoracic spine given that the rib head obscures part of the foramen and that the scapula limits that approach corridor. This approach is well suited for both calcified and soft disk herniations. The disk is typically approached from the side it is

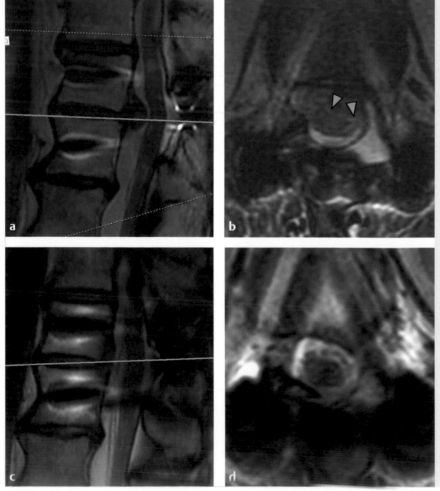

Fig. 19.1 Preoperative **(a)** sagittal and **(b)** axial T2-weighted MRI depicts a central T12/L1 disk protrusion with impingement of the spinal cord. *Green arrowheads* in **(b)** mark the border of the disk fragment. Postoperative **(c)** sagittal and **(d)** axial T2-weighted MRI confirms resection of the disk fragment and successful decompression of the spinal cord.

eccentric to. Disadvantages of this approach include a steep learning curve since the approach angle and intraoperative visualization are novel to traditionally trained spine surgeons. Moreover, additional bone work with resection of the superior articular process (SAP) is necessary to gain access into the spinal canal. For the novice, we recommend performing the foraminoplasty under vision rather than under fluoroscopic guidance to avoid inadvertent injury to the spinal cord. This approach is in particular useful for patients who have had a previous posterior approach or have pedicle screw–rod instrumentation as it may be performed avoiding scar tissue or removal of instrumentation.

19.2.1 Operating Room Setup and Patient Position

OR setup and patient position are described in detail in Chapter 6.

19.2.2 Approach

The approach corridor for a transforaminal endoscopic thoracic diskectomy aims directly toward the epidural space between the annulus of the index-level disk and the ventral thecal sac. For planning of the skin incision, an anteroposterior (AP) fluoroscopic endplate view of the caudal index-level vertebral body is obtained (▶ Fig. 19.2 **a**). The projection of the disk space is marked on the skin and the incision measured approximately 8 cm from the midline. Typically, the incision is in vicinity of the angle of the corresponding rib, which can easily be palpated. A small stab incision is produced and an 18-G needle/a Jamshidi needle is advanced medially along the projection of the disk space. Initially, care is taken that the needle is advanced along the outside of the ribs without entering the thoracic cavity. Approximately 2 cm lateral to the pedicle, the base of needle is elevated to allow the tip to pass ventral to the transverse process onto the lateral aspect of the caudal index-level SAP (*target area*). Using lateral fluoroscopy, the tip of the needle is "walked" ventrally along the lateral aspect of the SAP into the inferior aspect of the foramen (▶ Fig. 19.2 **a**). On AP X-ray, the needle is then advanced to the medial pedicle line. At that point, a lateral X-ray is obtained to make sure that the tip of needle is dorsal to the posterior vertebral line. Ascending size dilators are used to create a working corridor. Insertion of the dilators is carefully monitored on AP X-rays to avoid advancement beyond the medial pedicle line. Experienced surgeons may cautiously use bone trephines (TESSYS Access Kit, joimax) to create an approach corridor by partial resection of the rib head and ventral aspect of the SAP. However, bone reaming needs to be carried out focusing on bone resection by rotating the bone trephines with only minimal well-controlled forward pressure as unintended advancement into the spinal canal could cause catastrophic impingement of the thoracic spinal cord. Once the dilators have been placed, a beveled tubular working channel is introduced with the bevel facing the caudal pedicle. AP and lateral X-rays are obtained to confirm appropriate position of the tubular working cannel at the medial pedicle line and within the inferior aspect of the foramen (▶ Fig. 19.2 **b,c**).

19.3 Identify Bony Landmarks and Foraminoplasty

The dilators are removed, and the endoscope is brought into the tubular working channel. Connective tissue localized within the inferior portion of the intervertebral foramen is resected using grasper forceps and the bipolar cautery. The ventral surface of the SAP and the superior aspect of the caudal pedicle (*target area*) are exposed (▶ Fig. 19.3 **a**). A curved drill such as the Deflectable Shrill (joimax) or TipControl Articulating Burr (Wolf) may be used to resect the ventral aspect of the SAP and the superior portion of the caudal pedicle (▶ Fig. 19.3 **b**). For nonambiguous identification of the caudal pedicle, which constitutes the *principal anatomical landmark*, a Kerrison rongeur may be placed onto the rostral aspect of the pedicle and confirmed on AP X-ray.

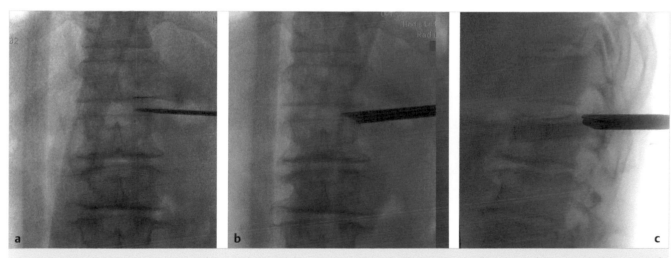

Fig. 19.2 Approach for a transforaminal endoscopic thoracic diskectomy as monitored with intraoperative fluoroscopy. **(a)** First, an endplate view of the caudal segment is obtained, and the disk projection is marked on the skin. **(b)** Following docking with the Jamshidi needle on the superior articular process (SAP; *target area*) and dilation of the working corridor, a tubular retractor is placed. **(c)** A final lateral X-ray confirms that the working channel is located in the intervertebral foramen dorsal to the posterior vertebral line.

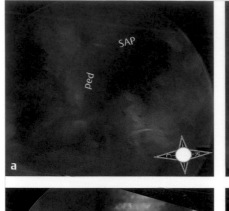
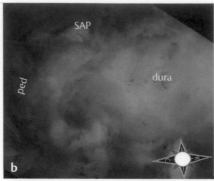
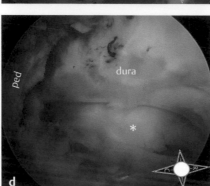

Fig. 19.3 Identify bony landmarks and prepare access to pathology. **(a)** Initial view of the rostral aspect of the pedicle (ped, *principal anatomical landmark*) and ventral surface of the superior articular process (SAP). **(b)** Using an articulating burr, additional bone of the superior aspect of the pedicle and the ventral aspect of the SAP are resected. The dura, typically covered by a layer of fat and connective tissue is identified medial to the caudal pedicle. **(c)** Using a blunt dissector, a plane between the thecal sac and disk herniation (*asterisk*) is developed. **(d)** Bone resection is continued until the rostrocaudal extent of the herniation is exposed.

19.3.1 Delineate Dura–Disk Interface

Depending on the degree of compression, various amounts of epidural fat are resected medial to the caudal pedicle using the grasping forceps and the bipolar cautery until the thecal sac is visualized. The dura is then followed ventrally and the plane between the thecal sac and the disk herniation is developed using blunt dissection with the bipolar cautery and blunt dissector (▶ Fig. 19.3 **c**). Once the disk herniation of the index level is visualized, additional resection of the SAP and caudal pedicle may be carried out if needed to gain access to the entire rostrocaudal extent of the disk herniation (▶ Fig. 19.3 **d**).

19.3.2 Resect Disk Herniation

The plane between the thecal sac and the disk herniation is developed using blunt dissection. The plane is easiest identified in the periphery of the disk herniation and then followed into the center. The bipolar cautery and the blunt dissector are useful tools to delineate the correct plane (▶ Fig. 19.4 **a**). Not infrequently, thoracic disk herniations are associated with ventral dural lacerations (see Chapter 25 for surgical management). Once the disk herniation is exposed, a combination of micro-

punches and burrs may be used to resect disk material (▶ Fig. 19.4 **b,c**). Once the middle of the lesion is reached, care must be taken not to violate the contralateral ventral dura as it drapes over the disk fragment and comes into view. Violation of the ventral dura is best avoided by identifying the correct plane in the periphery of the lesion and following into the epicenter of the compressive lesion. If compression is also caused by marginal osteophytes, they can be resected using an articulating burr (▶ Fig. 19.4 **d,e**). This maneuver is in particular useful in cases of heavily calcified central disk herniations; in these cases, partial resection of the adjacent vertebral bodies allows safe delivery of the disk fragment in a ventral direction away from the spinal cord.

19.4 Pearls and Pitfalls

- During advancement of the Jamshidi needle along the ribs, manually palpate the needle through the skin to confirm superficial passage (similar maneuver to passing a shunt catheter superficial to the clavicle).
- Bone reamers can be used to perform a foraminoplasty; however, limit the forward pressure in order to avoid

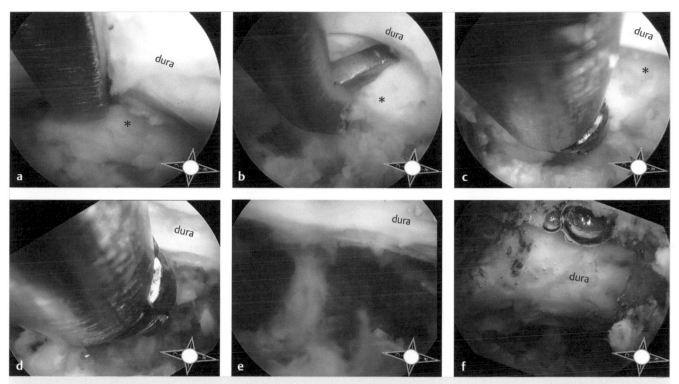

Fig. 19.4 Resection of the disk herniation. **(a)** The plane between dura and disk herniation (*asterisk*) is delineated using the blunt dissector. **(b)** Using an up-angled micro-punch, resection of the peripheral portion of the disk is initiated. **(c)** The calcified core of the disk is resected with the help of an articulating drill. **(d)** Once the disk herniation is removed, the marginal osteophytes of the adjacent endplates are resected using an articulating drill. **(e)** Following resection of the osteophytes and parts of the adjacent vertebral bodies and the disk, the ventral aspect of the thecal sac is decompressed. **(f)** Panoramic view of the decompressed thecal sac following the decompression.

inadvertent entry of the spinal canal and impingement of the spinal cord.
- Make sure to rule out ventral spinal cord herniation prior to performing an endoscopic transforaminal thoracic diskectomy.

- In cases of additional spinal cord compression by the posterior elements, decompress the posterior pathology first
- Utilize electrophysiological spinal cord monitoring for transforaminal endoscopic thoracic diskectomies.

Part 4

Cervical

20 Anterior Endoscopic Cervical Diskectomy

J. N. Alastair Gibson

20.1 Case Example

A 56-year-old ex-professional footballer presents with acute neck stiffness and pain radiating into the dorsum of his left forearm. He has found that his index finger is numb and feels that his grip strength has diminished. Examination reveals that he has approximately a 50% reduction in neck movement in all planes with a loss of biceps power and grip strength (4/5). His biceps reflex is also reduced on his left side. MR imaging confirms an acute cervical disk prolapse at C5/C6 with some minor reduction in disk space height with anterior osteophytic lipping on the vertebral margin (▶ Fig. 20.1). *The procedure performed is anterior endoscopic C5/C6 diskectomy.* The patient reports relief of his arm pain immediately following surgery but that it took 3 months for his grip strength to recover. One year after the procedure, he still experiences some mild neck stiffness on wakening from sleep but has no neck pain.

20.2 Indications

Anterior endoscopic spine surgery is appropriate for small to moderate posterior/posterolateral disk herniations and/or anterior foraminal compromise of the exiting nerve root at the affected level by disk or bony narrowing. The approach is not suited to foraminal compromise that is primarily posterior in nature in which case posterior endoscopic cervical foraminotomy is more appropriate (see Chapter 21). In the present clinical scenario, the patient had a history of trauma to his neck over several years and there was some evidence of minor spondylosis. Severe spondylosis with large osteophytes or segmental instability would preclude an anterior endoscopic approach. Disk space narrowing did not prevent a transdiskal approach, but sometimes distraction is necessary with a pinned (Caspar style) retractor, which requires a wider open exposure. If distraction is not possible, or a fragment is protruding cranially or

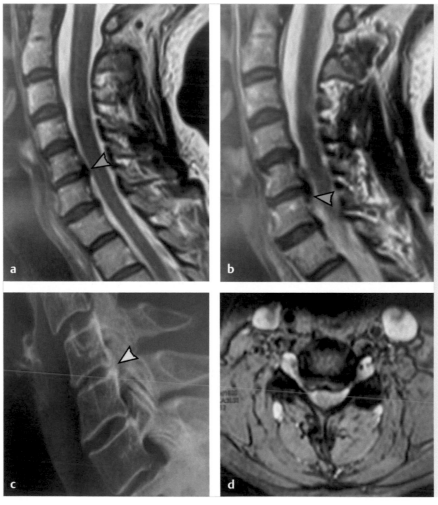

Fig. 20.1 (a) Preoperative MRI depicting a left C5/C6 disk herniation (*green arrowhead*). **(b)** There is a slight inferior extension on the left-side sagittal T2-weighted MRI (*green arrowhead*). **(c)** A lateral plain radiograph confirms the presence of minor osteophytic overgrowth (*yellow arrowhead*). **(d)** An axial T2-weighted MRI confirms the presence of some cord compression.

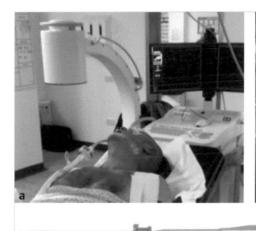
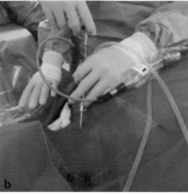

Fig. 20.2 (a) The patient is positioned with slight neck extension and with traction applied to the shoulders. (b) The instrumentation is brought in either completely percutaneously or via a short neck incision. (c) A cervical endoscope and working cannula (CESSYS, joimax GmbH) are coupled.

caudally behind either segmental vertebral body, then a transcorporeal approach or posterior endoscopic cervical diskectomy may provide better access. Indications for anterior endoscopic cervical diskectomy are the following:

- Contained posterior/posterolateral disk soft disk protrusions.
- Anterior foraminal compromise.
- As an adjunct to fusion/disk arthroplasty for severe disease at an adjacent level, where the surgeon wishes to avoid multilevel stabilization.

Operating room setup and patient positioning is shown in ▶ Fig. 20.2. The neck is extended, and the shoulders taped down. For the majority of patients, general anesthesia is required to avoid neck movement during the procedure. A selected few can tolerate analgo-sedation with a combination of subcutaneous lidocaine and intravenous remifentanil plus propofol.

20.3 Approach

The spine is approached percutaneously via a classical anterolateral neck incision. At the appropriate level, as identified by a radiograph, an 18-G needle is inserted to the margin of the disk between the carotid sheath laterally and the esophagus medially (▶ Fig. 20.2). It is safer to use a mini-open access (1.5-cm skin incision) to avoid injury to the carotid artery or any of the small thyroid venous branches. Aiming at the uncinate process (*target area*), the tip of the needle is advanced 50% across the disk under image intensifier guidance. The approach can either be an ipsilateral or a contralateral oblique as per the surgeon's choice and location of the disk protrusion. A guide wire is then inserted.

20.4 Tissue Dilation and Placement of Working Tube

Over the wire, 2 and 3-mm dilators are passed. Care should be taken not to advance the guidewire into the cord during insertion of the dilators by constantly visualizing depth of the instruments utilizing lateral fluoroscopic imaging. For lateral disk protrusions, it is usually also necessary to ream the margin of the uncinate process with a 3-mm cannulated reamer. A 4.8-mm-diameter working cannula may then be appropriately placed allowing introduction of the 3.9-mm endoscope connected to a high-definition camera. Constant irrigation facilitates the removal of disk fragments and provides tissue cooling.

20.5 Diskectomy

It is important to constantly check the position of the instruments on both anteroposterior and lateral fluoroscopic imaging (▶ Fig. 20.3). For foraminal herniations, the instrument positioning is viewed on a 45-degree oblique projection. Most commonly, disk material is removed in fragments. The posterior longitudinal ligament may be breached by tissue herniating into the canal that is extracted using a micro-punch or grasping forceps (▶ Fig. 20.4). Bleeding is rarely encountered.

20.6 Foraminotomy

Often, only minimal reaming is required to open the foramen adequately, but it is useful to have either a powered burr (Shrill, joimax GmbH) or side-cutting laser available.

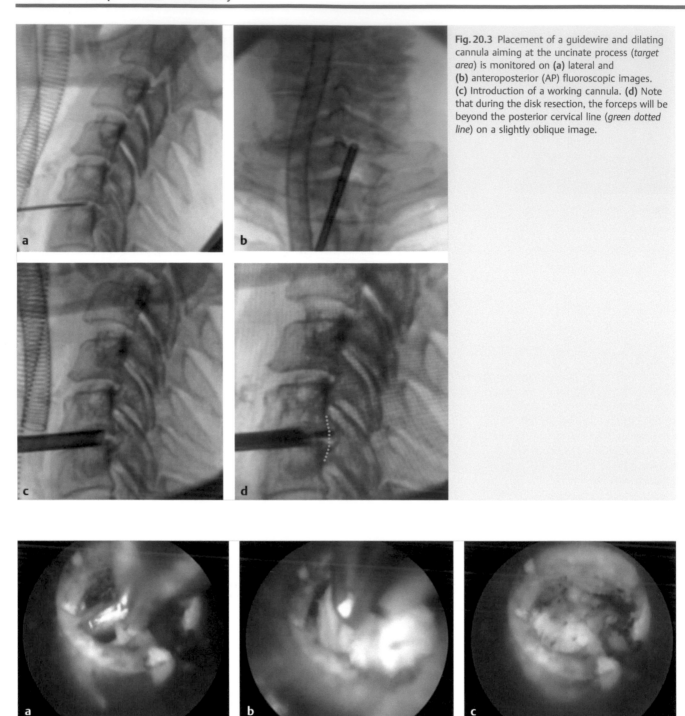

Fig. 20.3 Placement of a guidewire and dilating cannula aiming at the uncinate process (*target area*) is monitored on **(a)** lateral and **(b)** anteroposterior (AP) fluoroscopic images. **(c)** Introduction of a working cannula. **(d)** Note that during the disk resection, the forceps will be beyond the posterior cervical line (*green dotted line*) on a slightly oblique image.

Fig. 20.4 Endoscopic resection of disk fragments. **(a,b)** Utilizing cup forceps, the disk sequester is retrieved. **(c)** Inspection of the decompressed neural elements.

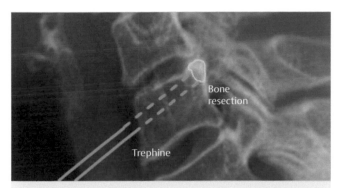

Fig. 20.5 Transcorporeal approach.

20.7 Pearls and Pitfalls

- Check and double-check the correct level of surgery (ensure the Atlas is visualized radiographically).
- Approach technique: For herniations cranial or caudal to the disk space, access via a transdiskal approach may be impossible. In this instance, it may be more appropriate to drill the vertebral body and place the working channel transcorporeal (▶ Fig. 20.5).
- Access to C2/C3 may be limited by the position of the mandible and should be avoided in "short-necked" patients.
- The cervical video endoscope is fragile due to its size. Care should be taken not to bend the scope and a second scope should be available in case of damage to the integral light fibers.
- Although not mandatory, cervical cord neuromonitoring provides an additional level of surgical safety. It is essential if any posterior ossification of the longitudinal ligament is present as the ligament is frequently adherent to the cord.

21 Posterior Endoscopic Cervical Foraminotomy

Christoph P. Hofstetter

21.1 Case Example

A 40-year old female surgeon presents with worsening neck, right arm pain, and weakness. The pain radiates into her proximal lateral right arm and is 4/10 in severity. On examination, the patient has right triceps (2/5) and hand pronation weakness (3/5). Preoperative cervical MRI reveals severe right C5/C6 and moderate right C6/C7 foraminal stenosis (▶ Fig. 21.1). *The procedures performed were right posterior endoscopic C5/C6 and C6/C7 foraminotomies.* Three months after the surgery, the patient has experienced a robust recovery of her neurologal function. Her right triceps has improved to 4+/5 and her pronation to 4/5. Her neck and upper extremity pain has resolved.

21.2 Indications

Posterior endoscopic cervical foraminotomies allow for effective decompression of cervical foraminal stenosis. The approach utilizes a traditional posterior interlaminar corridor similar to minimally invasive tubular surgery. Bone resection includes a small hemilaminotomy for localization of the thecal sac and the origin of the index-level nerve root. Resection of the facet joint is limited to approximately the medial one-third of the inferior articular process and the superior articular process (SAP) just beyond the lateral aspect of the caudal pedicle. The need for bone removal is typically less with endoscopic technique compared to minimally invasive surgery given that the endoscope provides off-axis panoramic visualization and can therefore look "around corners" rather than requiring a straight line of sight. Endoscopic posterior cervical foraminotomies are well suited to treat cervical foraminal stenosis caused by degenerative changes such as disk–osteophyte complexes, hypertrophic uncinate processes, or subluxation of the SAP.

If the foraminal stenosis is largely due to vertical foraminal stenosis (short pedicle–pedicle distance), a posterior cervical foraminotomy achieves only limited decompression even with partial resection of the rostral portion of the caudal pedicle. In these cases, an indirect foraminal decompression via an anterior cervical diskectomy and fusion should be considered. Endoscopic posterior foraminotomies are also well suited for the resection of lateral disk herniations. However, if the disk herniation extends medially beyond the lateral border of the spinal cord, an anterior procedure should be considered. In general, bilateral foraminal stenosis, additional central stenosis, or segmental dynamic instability should be addressed with more traditional anterior or posterior procedures. An exception to this rule are patients with unilateral foraminal stenosis and central stenosis mainly due to buckling of the yellow ligament; in these often-elderly patients, an endoscopic posterior cervical foraminotomy can be combined with a cervical unilateral laminotomy for bilateral decompression (see Chapter 21).

21.3 Approach

A carefully planned approach trajectory is extremely important for posterior endoscopic foraminotomies. An optimal rostrocaudal inclination of the approach trajectory minimizes the need for removal of rostral lamina and inferior articular process and allows for unobstructed access to the intervertebral foramen beyond the lateral aspect of the caudal index-level pedicle upon decompression. Moreover, the targeting technique proposed in the current chapter provides an easily reproducible and consistent view of the nerve root in relation to the bony anatomy. A consistent approach angle facilitates maneuvers for additional nerve root decompression such as resection of the rostral aspect of the caudal pedicle or access to the disk–osteophyte

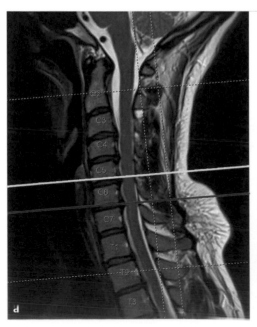
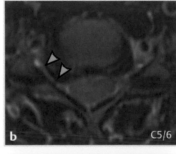
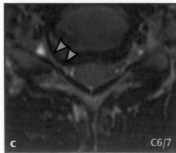

Fig. 21.1 Preoperative **(a)** sagittal and **(b,c)** axial T2-weighted MRI of the cervical spine depict multilevel mild central stenosis and severe right C5/C6 and C6/C7 foraminal stenosis (*green arrowheads*).

complex ventral to the nerve root. The surgery is carried out with the patient under general anesthesia, positioned on a radiolucent table in a prone position with the head secured in a Mayfield head holder. For planning of the skin incision, the ipsilateral medial pedicle line is marked on the skin using anteroposterior (AP) fluoroscopic imaging (▶ Fig. 21.2 **a**). Then obtaining a lateral X-ray, the trajectory of the index-level disk space and the facet joint are marked (▶ Fig. 21.2 **b,c**). The rostrocaudal approach trajectory is determined by splitting the angle of the disk space and facet joint in half (▶ Fig. 21.2 **d**). The skin incision is marked where the rostrocaudal approach trajectory intersects with the medial pedicle line. A small skin vertical incision is carried out with a no. 11 blade. Given the dense fascial layers of the neck muscles, it can be useful to sharply dissect the superficial fascial planes with the no. 11 blade. Then, a trocar is advanced carefully with small rostrocaudal movements along the determined approach trajectory. The rostrocaudal movements increase the size of leading edge, which facilitates detection of the edges of the lamia. This in

combination with lateral fluoroscopic guidance minimizes the risk of unintended advancement into the spinal canal. The goal is to palpate the juxtaposed edges of the index-level laminae, which serve as the *target area* of this approach. Under lateral fluoroscopic guidance, serial dilators are advanced with a rotational movement with only minimal well-controlled forward pressure as nonintended advancement into the spinal canal could cause catastrophic impingement of the thoracic spinal cord. Beveled dilators may be used to strip muscles off the lamina in order to facilitate the transition from palpation to visualization. At this point, an AP-X-ray should be obtained to confirm that the tip of the dilator is centered in vicinity of the medial pedicle line (▶ Fig. 21.2 **e**). The dilators should be kept in solid contact with the edge of the laminae by applying gentle downward pressure in order to minimize tissue creep. Following serial dilation, a 30-degree beveled working tube is placed with the open bevel facing medially. The edge of the lamina should be palpated with the bevel of the working tube, and then kept in solid bone contact while the endoscope is introduced.

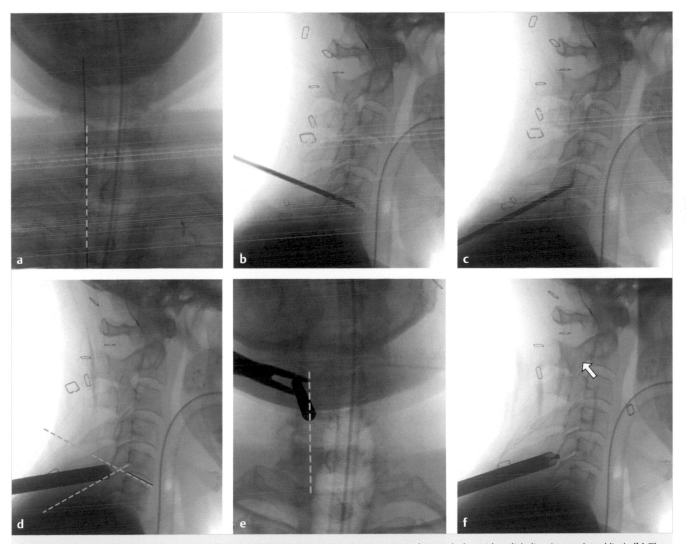

Fig. 21.2 Intraoperative fluoroscopic approach planning. **(a)** An anteroposterior X-ray is used to mark the mid-pedicle line (*green dotted line*). **(b)** The trajectory of the index-level disk space is marked on a lateral X-ray. **(c)** The trajectory of the facet joint is also marked. **(d)** The approach angle is determined by splitting the angle of the disk space and facet joint. The incision is marked where this line intersects with the medial pedicle line. The trocar and serial dilators are advanced. **(e)** The ideal docking place is between the juxtaposed margins of the index-level laminae (*target area*) centered on the mid-pedicle line. **(f)** The inferior edge of the rostral lamina is resected. A final confirmation of the level is obtained.

21.4 Identification of Bony Landmarks

First, the juxtaposed edges of the index-level laminae, which have been palpated with the dilators and bevel of the working tube, are visualized. To achieve this, overlying muscle and connective tissue are resected using the bipolar cautery and micro-punches. During this phase, the bevel of the tubular retractor may be used like a Cobb elevator to assist with dissection and retraction of soft tissue. The goal is to visualize the juxtaposed edges of the index-level laminae including their lateral "**V**"-shaped transition at the facet joint (*target area*; ▶ Fig. 21.3 **a**).

21.5 Hemilaminotomy

A small hemilaminotomy is carried out by resecting superior lamina along the bony attachment of the yellow ligament using a diamond burr (▶ Fig. 21.3 **b**). At this point, a final lateral X-ray may be obtained to confirm that the correct spinal level was targeted (▶ Fig. 21.2 **f**). The hemilaminotomy is completed by resecting the superior edge of the caudal lamina (▶ Fig. 21.3 **c**). Typically, the yellow ligament thins out quickly ventral to the inferior lamina and the epidural space becomes visible in the inferior portion of the hemilaminotomy. Upon careful

coagulation of epidural vessels, the yellow ligament is resected using a micro-punch and Kerrison rongeurs (▶ Fig. 21.3 **d**).

21.6 Identify the Index-Level Nerve Root

Once the hemilaminotomy is completed and the dura is exposed, additional bone and yellow ligament are resected laterally until the lateral margin of the thecal sac come into view (▶ Fig. 21.3 **d**). At this point, the index-level nerve root including its shoulder and axilla should be identified (▶ Fig. 21.3 **d**). The proximal nerve root is often traversed dorsally by a small ligament that is closely associated with the ventral surface of the SAP (▶ Fig. 21.3 **e**). This ligament may be elevated from the nerve root using a bunt dissector (▶ Fig. 21.3 **f**) and then resected with a Kerrison rongeur or micro-punch. This allows complete exposure of the nerve root.

21.7 Foraminal Decompression

Using a diamond burr, approximately the medial one-third of the inferior articular process is resected (▶ Fig. 21.4 **a**). Resection of the inferior articular process reveals the dorsal aspect of the SAP including the tip. Then the exposed SAP is resected

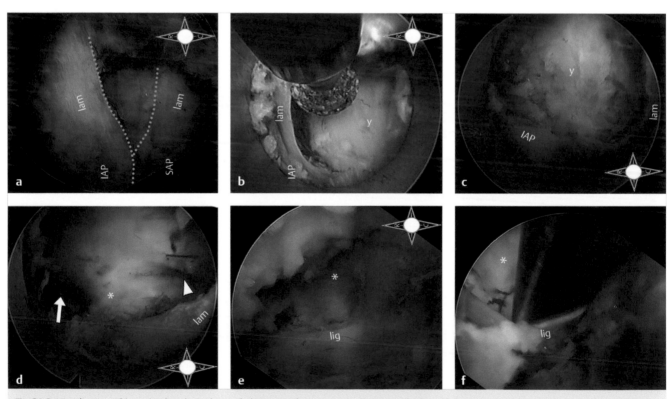

Fig. 21.3 Visualization of bony landmarks and neural elements. The *target area* (juxtaposed edges of the index-level laminae) is exposed. (a) The two edges form a "V"-shaped angle at the transition to the facet joint (*dotted green line*). (b) Using a high-speed drill, a hemilaminotomy of the inferior edge of the superior lamina is performed, which exposes the yellow ligament (y). Additional resection of the superior edge of the caudal lamina completes the hemilaminotomy. (c) Note how the yellow ligament thins out in the inferior portion of the hemilaminotomy site. (d) Following resection of the yellow ligament, the thecal sac and the shoulder (*arrow*) and axilla (*arrowhead*) of the index-level nerve root are exposed (*asterisk*). (e) The proximal nerve root is typically traversed dorsally by a small ligament (lig). (f) Elevating the ligament with a blunt dissector exposes the proximal aspect of the index-level nerve root (*asterisk*). Abbreviations: IAP, inferior articular process; lam, lamina; SAP, superior articular process.

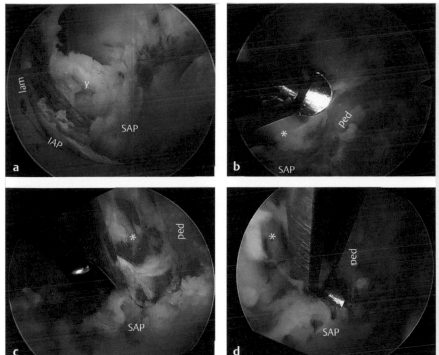

Fig. 21.4 Foraminal decompression. **(a)** Following resection of approximately the medial one-third of the inferior articular process (IAP), the superior articular process (SAP) comes into view. **(b)** Subsequent resection of the medial aspect of the SAP reveals the outline of the caudal index-level pedicle (ped; *principal anatomical landmark*) caudal to the nerve root (*asterisk*). **(c)** The rostral portion of the SAP is resected using a side-cutting burr. **(d)** The inferior aspect of the SAP rostral to the pedicle is undercut using a Kerrison rongeur. Abbreviation: y, yellow ligament.

using a diamond burr. Upon resection of the medial aspect of the SAP, the outline of the caudal pedicle that constitutes the *principal anatomical landmark* becomes visible (▶ Fig. 21.4 **b**). Using a Kerrison rongeur, the pedicle can be palpated. The nerve root is typically found just rostral to the pedicle. The SAP is resected until the lateral margin of the pedicle. Undercutting the SAP provides additional decompression of the nerve root comes into view. Undercutting is best started at the tip of the SAP using a small side-biting burr or small Kerrison rongeur (▶ Fig. 21.4 **c**). Importantly, the heel of the Kerrison rongeur is kept rostral to the nerve root to avoid compression of the nerve root during this maneuver. Once the rostral portion of the foramen is decompressed, the nerve root typically becomes more mobile, which allows for easier undercutting of the caudal portion of the SAP. The goal is to decompress the nerve root to the lateral aspect of the caudal pedicle

21.8 Optional Partial Caudal Pedicle Resection

Partial resection of the caudal pedicle may be useful if the nerve root continues to be compressed by the caudal pedicle following dorsal foraminal recompression. First, the nerve root is gently mobilized rostrally using a blunt dissector. Then a small side-protected side-cutting burr is utilized to resect the rostral one-third of the caudal pedicle (▶ Fig. 21.5 **a,b**). The configuration of the pedicle should be studied on preoperative imaging to avoid complete resection and possible destabilization of the segment. Also, the course of the vertebral artery should be studied to avoid injury of an aberrant vessel.

21.9 Optional Resection of Disk-Osteophyte Complex

The nerve root is gently mobilized rostrally. The bony component of the disk–osteophyte complex may be resected using a diamond burr or side-protected side-biting burr (▶ Fig. 21.5 **c**). Alternatively, small hand-driven bone trephines may be used. Residual bone and soft tissue may be further mobilized using a blunt dissector or curette. A micro-punch is useful for resection of fibrous tissue such as annulus (▶ Fig. 21.5 **d**). Small up-angled cup forceps are very helpful to retrieve fragments localized ventral to the nerve root.

21.10 Pearls and Pitfalls

- Counting the spinal levels on lateral fluoroscopic images can be challenging in the lower cervical spine since the spine is obscured by the shoulder girdle. Utilizing AP X-rays can be helpful, counting segments upward from T1. Intraoperative navigation is a useful technology to assist with identification of the correct level and planning of the trajectory (see Chapter 4).
- The muscle fascial planes can be difficult to penetrate during the initial tissue dilation. One strategy is to advance a no. 11 blade with small rostrocaudal movements (2–3 mm at the tip) to cut fascia under lateral fluoroscopic control.
- As with other interlaminar approaches, choosing the approach trajectory determines the view of the exposed anatomy and structures that can be reached. Choosing a too steep rostrocaudal approach angle hampers exposure of the

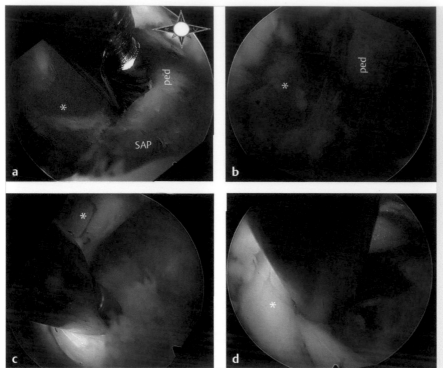

Fig. 21.5 Optional maneuvers for nerve root decompression. **(a)** Utilizing a small side-cutting burr, the rostral aspect of the caudal pedicle (ped) may be resected in order to provide additional decompression of the nerve root (*asterisk*). **(b)** The nerve root is decompressed beyond the lateral aspect of the pedicle. Disk–osteophyte complexes ventral to the nerve root (*asterisk*) may be addressed via the caudal circumference of the nerve root utilizing **(c)** small side-cutting burrs or **(d)** micro-punches. Abbreviation: SAP, superior articular process.

nerve root as it is behind the pedicle and the endoscope is deflected by the caudal lamina and pedicle. Choosing a too flat approach angle in line with the disk space requires more resection of the rostral index-level lamina and inferior articular process to reach the foramen.

- Patients with large disk–osteophyte complexes might benefit from the use of electrophysiological monitoring. Monitoring spontaneous electromyographic (EMG) activity helps minimize irritation of the nerve root during retraction resection of the disk–osteophyte complex.

22 Cervical Endoscopic Unilateral Laminotomy for Bilateral Decompression

Daniel Carr and Christoph P. Hofstetter

22.1 Case Example

An 84-year-old man with a history of lung cancer presents with progressive loss of upper extremity dexterity and gait unsteadiness. On examination, the patient has decreased bilateral upper extremity intrinsic muscle strength (4/5), bilateral positive Babinski signs, and displays unsteady-gait requiring a walker. The patient has a kyphotic posture with thoracolumbar kyphosis and compensatory cervical lordosis (▶ Fig. 22.1 **a**). Preoperative cervical MRI reveals severe C2/C3 and moderate C3/C 4 spinal stenosis (▶ Fig. 22.1 **b**). *The procedures performed were C2/C3 and C3/C4 endoscopic unilateral laminotomies for bilateral decompression (ULBD).* Intraoperative CT scan reveals adequate decompression of the posterior bony elements at C2/C3 and C3/C4 (▶ Fig. 22.2 **a**). A postoperative MRI depicts sufficient decompression of the spinal cord at C2/C3 and C3/C4 (▶ Fig. 22.2 **b**). After 3 months, the patient's neurological examination has improved. His hand intrinsic strength has increased to 4+/5. Moreover, his myelopathy has improved, and his Babinski's signs are negative bilaterally. The patient is now able to ambulate with a cane.

22.2 Indications

Cervical endoscopic ULBD allows for decompression of the spinal canal in cases of cervical spinal stenosis caused by the dorsal elements. This type of pathology is commonly found in the cervical spine of elderly patients (> 80 years) who compensate for thoracolumbar kyphosis with hyperextension of their neck. This compensatory cervical "hyper-lordosis" causes buckling of the yellow ligament, with stenosis in the upper cervical levels. Given the advanced age and commonly vast amount of comorbidities, these patients are typically not candidates for traditional reconstructive surgeries addressing both the deformity and spinal stenosis. Endoscopic ULBD utilizes a traditional posterior interlaminar corridor similar to minimally invasive tubular surgery. Bone resection includes an ipsilateral hemilaminotomy, generous undercutting of the juxtaposed spinous processes, and contralateral decompression. Cervical endoscopic ULBD is not indicated for patients with spinal stenosis due to dynamic segmental instability or stenosis caused by anterior pathology such as disc bulges, osteophytes, or kyphosis.

22.3 Approach

A carefully planned approach trajectory is extremely important for endoscopic ULBD. An optimal rostrocaudal inclination of the approach trajectory minimizes the need for bone removal and allows for adequate contralateral access with undercutting of the juxtaposed spinous processes. The patient is under general anesthesia and positioned prone on a radiolucent table with the head secured in a Mayfield head holder. For planning of the skin incision, the projection of the ipsilateral medial pedicle line is marked on the skin utilizing anteroposterior (AP) fluoroscopic imaging (▶ Fig. 22.3 **a**). Then a true lateral fluoroscopic image of the index level is obtained. The approach trajectory is constructed by connecting the posterior aspect of the index-level disk space with a line between the index-level spinous processes and marked on the skin (▶ Fig. 22.3 **b**). The skin incision is marked where the approach trajectory intersects with

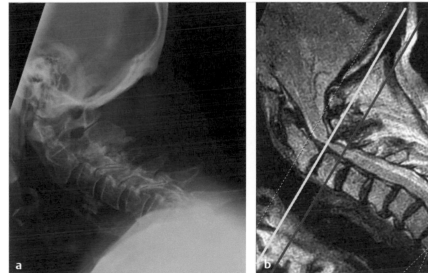
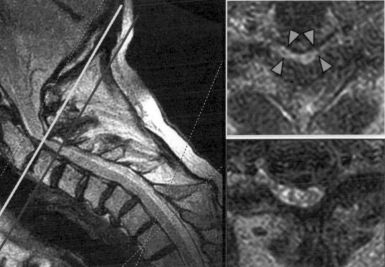

Fig. 22.1 (a) Preoperative lateral X-ray depicts thoracic kyphosis with compensatory upper cervical lordosis. (b) Sagittal T2-weighted MRI reveals severe stenosis at C2/C3 and C3/C4. The upper panel shows an axial T2-weighted image of the C2/C3 level. The green arrowheads delineate the circumference of the compressed spinal cord. The lower panel shows an axial image of the spinal cord at C3/C4.

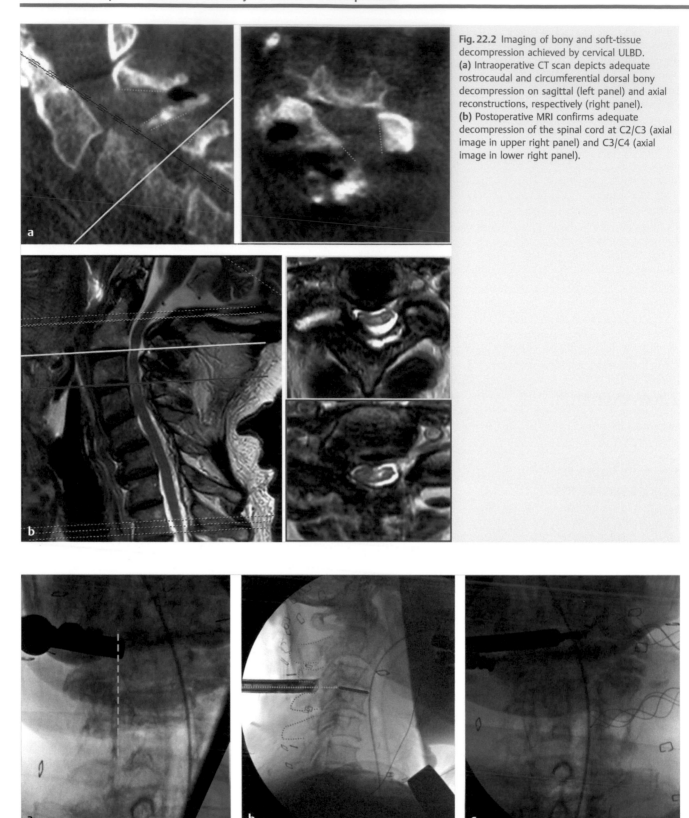

Fig. 22.2 Imaging of bony and soft-tissue decompression achieved by cervical ULBD. **(a)** Intraoperative CT scan depicts adequate rostrocaudal and circumferential dorsal bony decompression on sagittal (left panel) and axial reconstructions, respectively (right panel). **(b)** Postoperative MRI confirms adequate decompression of the spinal cord at C2/C3 (axial image in upper right panel) and C3/C4 (axial image in lower right panel).

Fig. 22.3 Intraoperative fluoroscopic approach planning. **(a)** Anteroposterior (AP) X-ray confirms the location of the tip of the working cannula in vicinity of the medial pedicle line. **(b)** Lateral X-ray demonstrates the approach trajectory (*green dotted line*) between the index-level spinous processes (*blue dotted line*) aiming at the posterior aspect of the disk space (*red line*). **(c)** AP X-ray confirms the adequate extent of the contralateral decompression.

the mid-pedicle line. A small vertical skin incision is carried out with a no. 11 blade. Given the dense fascial layers of the neck muscles, it is often necessary to sharply dissect the fascial planes with a no. 11 blade under lateral fluoroscopic guidance. Serial dilators are then advanced with small rostrocaudal movements along the determined approach trajectory. Both the rostrocaudal movement of the dilators and lateral fluoroscopic guidance are utilized to prevent unintended advancement of the dilators into the spinal canal. The goal is to palpate the juxtaposed edges of the index-level laminae, which constitute the target area of this approach. Beveled dilators may be used to strip muscles off the lamina in order to facilitate the transition from palpation to visualization of the target area. At this point, an AP X-ray should be obtained to confirm that the tip of the dilator is centered in vicinity of the medial pedicle line (▶ Fig. 22.3 **a**). Attention should be paid to keep the dilators in solid contact with the edge of the laminae by applying gentle controlled downward pressure. Following serial dilation, a 30-degree beveled working tube is placed with the opening facing medially. The edge of the lamina should be palpated with the bevel of the working tube, and then kept in solid bone contact by applying gentle downward pressure while the endoscope is introduced.

22.4 Visualizing Target Area

First, the juxtaposed edges of the rostral and caudal laminae, which have been palpated with the dilators and bevel of the working tube, are visualized. To achieve this, overlying muscle and connective tissue are resected using the bipolar cautery and micro-punches. During this phase, the bevel of the tubular retractor may be used as a Cobb elevator to assist with dissection and retraction of soft tissue. The goal is to visualize the juxtaposed edges of the index-level laminae, which constitute the *target area* of this approach (▶ Fig. 22.4 **a**). The lamina edges should be exposed spanning from spinous process medially and to the "V" of the facet joint laterally.

22.5 Hemilaminotomy

Using a diamond burr, a hemilaminotomy of the superior lamina along the bony attachment of the yellow ligament is carried out (▶ Fig. 22.4 **b**). The lamina insertion of the yellow ligament is considered the *principal anatomical landmark* of this approach as it guides the entire bony decompression. At this point, a final lateral X-ray may be obtained to confirm that the correct spinal level was targeted. The hemilaminotomy is completed by resecting the superior edge of the inferior lamina (▶ Fig. 22.4 **c**). Typically, the yellow ligament thins out ventral to the inferior lamina and the epidural space becomes visible in the inferior portion of the hemilaminotomy. Upon careful coagulation of epidural vessels, the yellow ligament is resected using a micro-punch and Kerrison rongeur (▶ Fig. 22.3 **d**). The edges of the lamina are carefully undercut using Kerrison rongeurs (▶ Fig. 22.4 **e**). Identification of the ipsilateral margin of the thecal sac concludes the ipsilateral decompression (▶ Fig. 22.4 **f**).

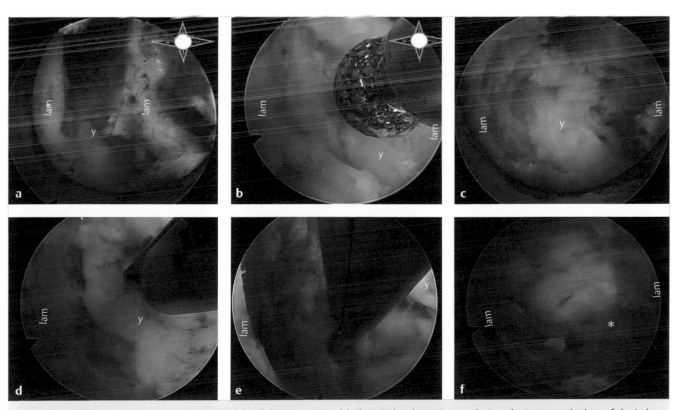

Fig. 22.4 Identification of bony landmarks and ipsilateral decompression. (a) The initial endoscopic view depicts the juxtaposed edges of the index-level laminae (lam) with yellow ligament (y) in between. (b) The hemilaminotomy is initiated by drilling along the inferior edge of the rostral lamina. Once the hemilaminotomy is partially completed, yellow ligament is seen in the rostral aspect. (c) In the caudal aspect, the yellow ligament is thinned out and allows the view of the epidural space. (d) The yellow ligament and (e) the bony edges are resected piecemeal using the Kerrison rongeur. (f) Completed ipsilateral decompression of the thecal sac. The *asterisk* marks the origin of the ipsilateral index-level nerve root.

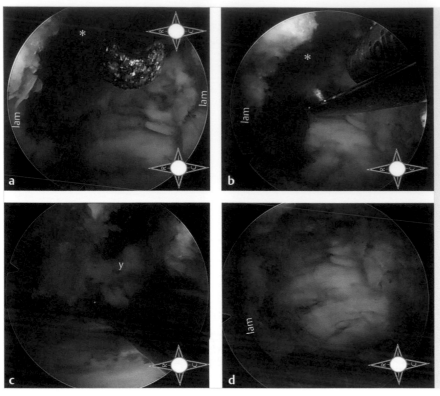

Fig. 22.5 Undercutting the spinous process and contralateral decompression. The base of the rostral spinous process (*asterisk*) is generously undercut using **(a)** the diamond burr and **(b)** the Kerrison rongeur. Bulging contralateral yellow ligament is resected with the Kerrison rongeur. **(c)** During this maneuver, greatest caution is taken not to compress the spinal cord. **(d)** A final view of the entirely decompressed spinal cord is depicted. Abbreviation: lam, lamina.

22.6 Undercutting the Spinous Process

Generous undercutting of the spinous processes is imperative in order to avoid impingement of the spinal cord during the contralateral decompression. Using a diamond burr, the ipsilateral hemilaminotomy is extended medially into the base of the adjacent spinous processes. Importantly, during the process of undercutting the spinous process, superficial overhanging bone needs to be constantly resected in order to allow a straight unobstructed access to the contralateral side. Thus, a generous wedge-shaped portion of the base of the spinous process is resected in order to allow access to the contralateral side without exerting any pressure onto the spinal cord (▶ Fig. 22.2 **a** and ▶ Fig. 22.5 **a**). Typically, the juxtaposed aspects of the index-level spinous processes need to be undercut in order to decompress the central portion of the spinal canal as well as to gain unobstructed access to the contralateral side.

22.7 Contralateral Decompression

Undercutting of the contralateral lamina is carried out utilizing a side-cutting burr or Kerrison rongeur (▶ Fig. 22.5 **b**). If the contralateral lamina cannot be reached, additional undercutting of the spinous process needs to be performed. Any pressure onto the spinal cord must be avoided and electrophysiological monitoring should be carried out to confirm spinal cord function. The contralateral buckling yellow ligament is resected using a Kerrison rongeur (▶ Fig. 22.5 **c**). Once the contralateral thecal sac appeared decompressed, AP X-ray may be obtained to confirm the adequate extent of contralateral decompression

(▶ Fig. 22.2 **c**). At this point, complete decompression dorsal circumference of the cervical spine has been accomplished (▶ Fig. 22.5 **d**).

22.8 Pearls and Pitfalls

- Case selection: Endoscopic cervical ULBD will only treat cervical spinal stenosis caused by posterior pathology such as buckling of the yellow ligament.
- Choice of appropriate endoscope: Small-diameter (iLESSYS Pro [joimax] or interlaminar endoscope [Wolf]) versus larger-diameter endoscope (iLESSYS delta, [joimax] or central stenosis endoscope [Wolf]). Both types of scopes may be used. The smaller-diameter scope has the advantage of easier tissue dilation and easier transition from palpation to visualization of bony landmarks (given the smaller diameter of the working tube and less soft-tissue creep). The larger endoscope has the advantage to allow for the use of larger instruments and the larger working tube is less likely unintendedly advanced into the spinal canal given that the laminotomy defect is smaller than the diameter of the working tube.
- Counting the spinal levels on lateral fluoroscopic images can be challenging in the lower cervical spine since the spine is obscured by the shoulder girdle. Utilizing AP X-rays can be helpful with counting up from T1. Image navigation helps with planning and performing the approach (see Chapter 4).
- The muscle fascial planes can be difficult to penetrate during the initial tissue dilation. One strategy is to advance a no. 11 blade with small rostrocaudal movements (2–3 mm at the tip) to cut fascia under lateral fluoroscopic control.

- Always bring in instruments with the working channel pointing at bone to avoid unintended trauma to neural elements. Avoid using instruments with different shaft lengths.
- Always be aware of the position of the working tube to avoid compression of the spinal cord.
- The use of electrophysiological monitoring of the spinal cord function is strongly advised, in particular during contralateral decompression.

- Use the lowest irrigation pressure which still allows for a clear visualization and leave the yellow ligament in place during the bony decompression in order to minimize pressure onto the spinal cord. This is in particular important in stenosis cases with some ventral pathology such as a disc bulge.

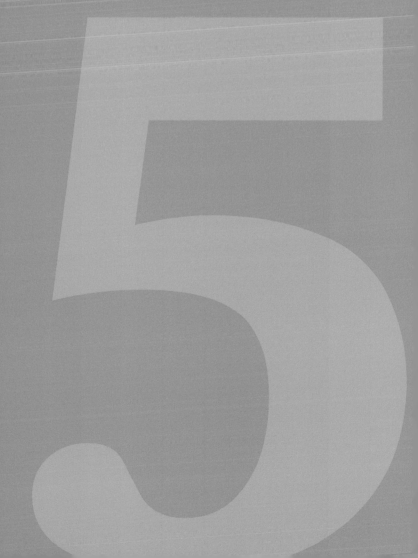

Part 5

Additional Topics

23 Adapting Full-Endoscopic Technique for Challenging Cases

Christoph P. Hofstetter

23.1 Morbidly Obese Patients

As long as the endoscope can reach the pathology, full-endoscopic spine surgery is only minimally affected by the subcutaneous fat pannus. For interlaminar approaches, the length of the tubular retractor is typically sufficient. For transforaminal approaches, a tubular retractor paired with a standard endoscope is sometimes too short. Most companies have extra-long endoscopes available if necessary (see Chapter 5). The necessary length of the tubular retractor can typically be determined on preoperative imaging. In morbidly obese patients, other issues such as maximum patient weight limit of the OR table, special padding, and increased medical risks need to be considered.

23.1.1 Case Example

A 57-year-old morbidly obese male (BMI 60) patient presented to our office with complaints of left lower extremity pain (10/10) and progressive left lower extremity weakness (dorsiflexion: 1/5; extensor hallucis longus [EHL]: 0/5; plantar flexion: 4/5). The patient had also sustained several falls and noted worsening bladder function. Preoperative MRI of the lumbar spine revealed multilevel spinal stenosis at L1/L2, L2/L3, L4/L5, and L5/S1 in the setting of a congenitally narrow spinal canal. The patient underwent endoscopic L1/L2, L2/L3, L4/L5, and L5/S1 unilateral laminotomies for bilateral decompression. He tolerated the procedure well. At his 12-month follow-up visit, his left lower extremity strength had improved (left dorsiflexion: 4/5; EHL: 3/5). He rated is left lower extremity pain as 4/10. The patient has lost 80 lb, is currently working full time, and ambulates without a cane (▶ Fig. 23.1).

23.1.2 Pearls and Pitfalls

- Full-endoscopic spine surgery is a well-suited technique for decompressive surgery in morbidly obese patients.
- Contralateral decompression during unilateral laminotomy for bilateral decompression (ULBD) may be hampered by the overlying soft tissue. Selecting a slightly more lateral incision facilitates reaching the contralateral recess.
- The length of the surgical corridor should be measured on preoperative imaging to make sure that the tubular retractor reaches the target area.

23.2 Adapting the Transforaminal Approach for Caudally Migrated Disk Herniations

Several modifications allow us to utilize the transforaminal approach for resection of caudally migrated disk herniations. Choosing a steeper trans-isthmus approach trajectory helps gain access to disk herniations behind the superior half of the caudal index-level pedicle (*zone 3*; ▶ Fig. 23.2).[1] Once the disk herniation extends into zone 4, partial resection of the superior portion of the pedicle is necessary. A steep trans-isthmus approach trajectory in combination with partial resection of the superior portion of the caudal index-level pedicle allows us to resect disk fragments from zone 4.

23.2.1 Case Example

A 33-year-old woman presents with a 4-year history of right lower extremity radiating pain. The patient describes the pain as radiating from her lower back to the lateral thigh and posterolateral calf and rates it as 3/10 in severity. On examination, the patient has right gluteus medius weakness (4/5) and plantar flexion weakness (4/5). A Preoperative MRI depicts a right L4/L5 disk herniation with downward migration and impingement of the right L5 and S1 nerve root (▶ Fig. 23.3 **a,b**). The patient underwent a right transforaminal endoscopic L4/L5 diskectomy with trans-isthmus approach and resection of the rostral portion of the left L5 pedicle (▶ Fig. 23.3 **c,d**). During the procedure, the medial aspect of the L5 pedicle served as the principal anatomical landmark (▶ Fig. 23.3 **e**). The traversing L5 nerve root was localized just medial to the pedicle. Utilizing blunt and sharp dissection, the nerve root was dissected off the disk fragment, which was then retrieved using the grasping forceps (▶ Fig. 23.3 **f**). The patient tolerated the procedure well, had transient postoperative paresthesias in her L5 distribution, and was asymptomatic at her 2-week follow-up appointment.

23.2.2 Pearls and Pitfalls

- The transforaminal approach with a trans-isthmus trajectory and partial resection of the rostral portion of the caudal index-level pedicle allows for resection of zone 4 migrated disk fragments.
- The traversing nerve root is sometimes found lateral to the disk fragment. Entry into the spinal canal should be performed using continuous visualization to avoid damage to the neural structures.

23.3 Adapting the Transforaminal Approach for Rostrally Migrated Disk Herniations

The trans-superior articular process (trans-SAP) approach utilizing an approach trajectory in line with the disk space, docking on the SAP, and partial resection of the SAP allows for resection of zone 1 and 2 migrated disk fragments. Utilizing off-axis instruments such as semi-flexible grasper forceps greatly facilitate retrieval of rostrally migrated disk fragments. Retrieving rostrally migrated fragments at L5/S1 is technically challenging given the iliac crest.

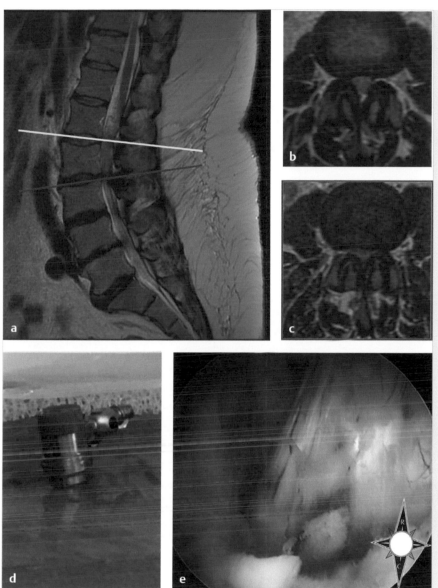

Fig. 23.1 Decompression surgery in morbidly obese patient. (a) Preoperative sagittal T2-weighted MRI depicts multilevel spinal stenosis, in particular at (b) L1/L2 and (c) L2/L3. (d) The 14-cm-long tubular retractor sufficient to reach the pathology. (e) Intraoperative image of decompressed neural elements.

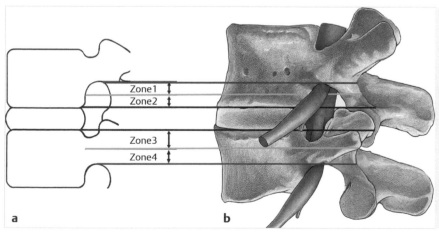

Fig. 23.2 Classification for migrated disk herniations for the transforaminal approach. (a,b) Disk migration is classified into four zones based on the direction and distance from the disk space: zone 1 (far up), zone 2 (near up), zone 3 (near down), and zone 4 (far down). (Adapted from Lee et al 2007.[1])

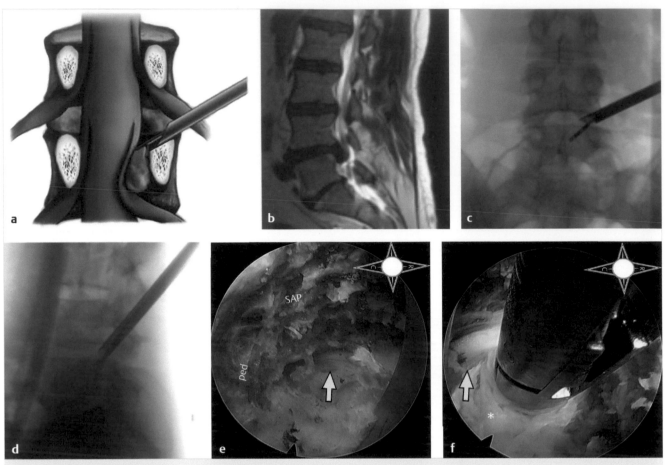

Fig. 23.3 Resection of caudally migrated disk fragment. **(a)** Illustration depicting the approach trajectory and partial resection of caudal index-level pedicle. **(b)** Sagittal MRI depicting an L4/L5 caudally migrated disk fragment. **(c)** Anteroposterior intraoperative fluoroscopic image depicting adequate reach. **(d)** Lateral intraoperative fluoroscopic image shows the trans-isthmus approach trajectory. **(e)** Intraoperative image of the rostral portion of the partially resected pedicle (ped) and the traversing nerve root (*arrow*) medial to the landmark. **(f)** Following dissection of the nerve root, the disk fragment (*asterisk*) is carefully retrieved using the alligator technique. Abbreviation: SAP, superior articular process.

23.3.1 Case Example

A 57-year-old man presents with a 6-year history of left lower extremity pain. The pain radiates from his lower back to his lateral thigh and calf and is 8/10 in severity. On examination, the patient has left foot dorsiflexion (3/5), left EHL (1/5), and left gluteus medius (2/5) weakness. A preoperative MRI depicted left L4/L5 rostrally migrated disk fragment (▶ Fig. 23.4 **a,b**). The patient underwent a left L4/L5 trans-SAP approach for resection of the disk fragment. Intraoperatively, the disk fragment was immediately encountered following the trans-SAP approach (▶ Fig. 23.4 **c,d**). The fragment was dissected off the traversing nerve root in a caudal-to-cranial fashion starting at the medial aspect of the caudal pedicle (▶ Fig. 23.4 **e**). Upon retrieval of the fragment, the exiting nerve descended onto the foramen (▶ Fig. 23.4 **f**). The patient tolerated the procedure well and his symptoms resolved.

23.3.2 Pearls and Pitfalls

- The trans-SAP approach allows retrieval of zone 2 and most zone 1 migrated disk herniations

- Partial resection of the SAP is necessary to gain entry into the canal when utilizing a rostral approach trajectory.

23.4 Resection of Synovial Cysts

Resection of synovial cysts is a great indication for full-endoscopic spine surgery. Both interlaminar and transforaminal approaches allow for resection of synovial cysts. Similar to traditional surgery, the dura should always be visualized first before the synovial cyst is addressed. If the synovial cyst is entered during the approach, the entry point into the spinal canal should be changed and additional bone resected if necessary in order to visualize the thecal sac. Synovial cysts often greatly deform the dura by creating folds and duplications (▶ Fig. 23.5 **c**). High-definition visualization offered by full-endoscopic spine surgery allows exploration of these dural folds and helps avoid dural lacerations. Synovial cysts are sometimes tightly adherent to the dura. Sharp dissection can be carried out using the sharp dissector, micro-scissors, or micro-punch. If dissection is not safely possible, adherent cyst wall may be left in place. The medial aspect of the facet joint giving rise to the cyst should be trimmed along the entire rostrocaudal

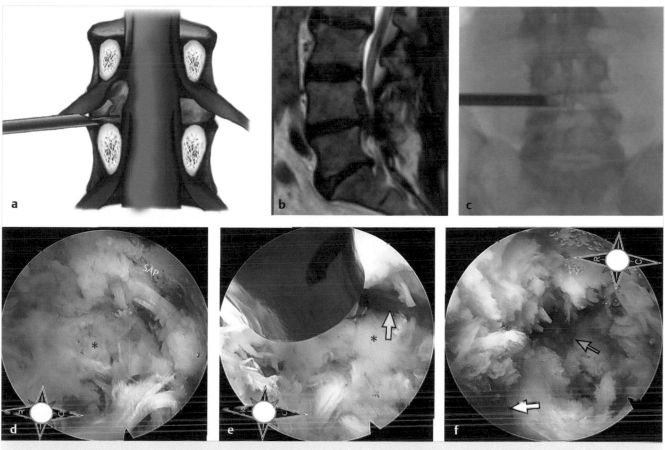

Fig. 23.4 Resection of rostrally migrated disk fragment. **(a)** Illustration and **(b)** T2-weighted MRI depicting a rostrally migrated L4/L5 disk herniation. **(c)** Intraoperative fluoroscopic images confirm rostral reach with the curved cautery probe. **(d)** Initial intraoperative view of the disk fragment (*asterisk*). **(e)** Starting at the rostral edge of the caudal pedicle, the traversing nerve root (*arrow*) is dissected off the disk fragment (*asterisk*). **(f)** Following resection of the fragment, the inferior endplate of L4 (*green arrow*) is visible and the exiting nerve root (*white arrow*) descends into the foramen. Abbreviation: SAP, superior articular process.

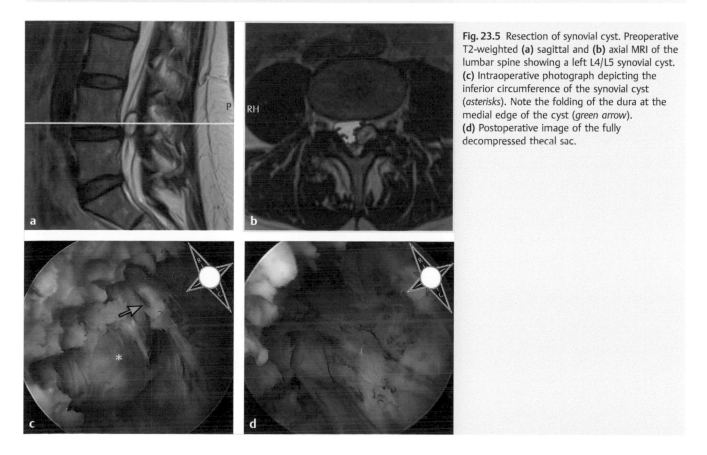

Fig. 23.5 Resection of synovial cyst. Preoperative T2-weighted **(a)** sagittal and **(b)** axial MRI of the lumbar spine showing a left L4/L5 synovial cyst. **(c)** Intraoperative photograph depicting the inferior circumference of the synovial cyst (*asterisks*). Note the folding of the dura at the medial edge of the cyst (*green arrow*). **(d)** Postoperative image of the fully decompressed thecal sac.

extent using a high-speed burr and the synovia resected in order to avoid recurrence.

23.4.1 Case Example

A 54-year-old woman presents with a 3-month history of left lower extremity radicular pain. She rates her pain as 10/10 in severity. On examination, she had left gluteus medius (2/5) and left EHL weakness (3/5). A preoperative MRI revealed a large left L4/L5 synovial cyst (▶ Fig. 23.5 **a,b**) with impingement of the traversing L5 nerve root. The patient underwent an inter-laminar endoscopic lateral recess decompression with resection of the synovial cyst. The dura was identified first and the inter-face with the cyst was carefully exposed (▶ Fig. 23.5 **c**). Using the elevator and the sharp dissector, the synovial cyst was dis-sected off the dura. A complete resection was achieved (▶ Fig. 23.5 **d**). The patient tolerated the procedure well and remains asymptomatic 3 years following the procedure.

23.4.2 Pearls and Pitfalls

- Synovial cysts are not an absolute indication for arthrodesis surgery.
- Synovial cysts are amenable to resection using the full-endoscopic technique.
- High-definition visualization allows us to recognize synovial cyst-related folding and duplications of the dura and thus preserve its integrity.

23.5 Transforaminal Access to L5/S1 in Patients with a High Iliac Crest

The transforaminal approach at L5/S1 is regarded as challenging in particular due to the iliac crest, a narrow foramen, and the great width of the L5/S1 facet joint. Moreover, the dorsal root ganglion of L5 is almost always located within the neurofora-men and fills more than 50% of the diameter.[2] Irritation of the L5 nerve root may lead to paresthesias or complex regional pain syndromes. For all these reasons, transforaminal approaches can be challenging at L5/S1 and should be planned and executed carefully. Several strategies are available to minimize L5 nerve root injury during L5/S1 approaches:

- Perform a trans-SAP approach, particularly in the cases where the iliac crest is projected above the mid-L5 pedicle[3] (for technique, see Chapter 17).
- Perform the case with the patient awake or with neuromonitoring.
- Minimize the duration of the intraforaminal work.
- Perform an interlaminar contralateral endoscopic lumbar foraminotomy instead, particularly in the cases with medial foraminal stenosis.
- Perform indirect decompression utilizing interbody spacers for cases of vertical foraminal stenosis (foraminal height < 10 mm).
- Utilize the interlaminar approach for pathology within the spinal canal.

23.5.1 Case Example

A 52-year-old woman with a surgical history of a right L4/L5 and L5/S1 interlaminar endoscopic lumbar lateral recess decompression 2 years prior presents with recurrent right lower extremity pain. Her pain started after a trip with exten-sive walking and follows an L5 distribution. She is neurologi-cally intact. An MRI of the lumbar spine reveals a right L5/S1 foraminal synovial cyst (▶ Fig. 23.6 **a**). The patient underwent a diagnostic right L5 block, which gave her complete transient relief. She underwent a right transforaminal endoscopic L5/S1 foraminotomy with resection of the foraminal synovial cyst. The foraminotomy was performed using a trans-SAP technique utilizing the medial aspect of the S1 pedicle as the principal anatomical landmark (▶ Fig. 23.6 **b**). The ventral aspect of the SAP and the lateral synovial capsule of the facet joint were resected (▶ Fig. 23.6 **c**). The extraforaminal yellow ligament was resected and the L5 nerve root entirely decompressed (▶ Fig. 23.6 **d**). The patient tolerated the procedure well and her right lower extremity pain has completely resolved 6 months after the procedure.

23.5.2 Pearls and Pitfalls

- Foraminal pathology at L5/S1 may be addressed using the trans-SAP approach (for technique, see Chapter 17).

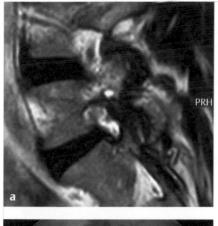
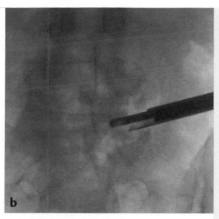
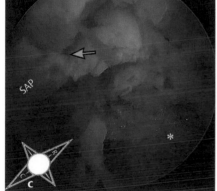
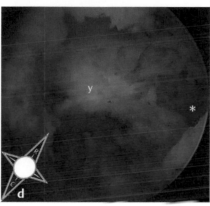

Fig. 23.6 L5/S1 foraminal synovial cyst. **(a)** Preoperative MRI depicts a synovial cyst in the lateral portion of the L5/S1 facet joint. **(b)** Intraoperative fluoroscopic confirmation of the S1 pedicle. **(c)** Exposure of the lateral aspect of the L5/S1 facet join. The extraforaminal aspect of the L5 nerve root is seen (*asterisk*). **(d)** Upon partial resection of the superior articular process (SAP), the L5 nerve root is decompressed (*asterisk*). Residual extraforaminal yellow ligament (y) is noted.

- For vertical foraminal stenosis at L5/S1, in particular with segmental coronal deformity, indirect decompression with an interbody cage and segmental arthrodesis should always be considered.
- Pathology within the spinal canal may be preferentially addressed using the interlaminar technique.
- The utility of the transforaminal approach may be limited at L5/S1, in particular with a steep pelvic crest.

References

[1] Lee S, Kim SK, Lee SH, et al. Percutaneous endoscopic lumbar discectomy for migrated disc herniation: classification of disc migration and surgical approaches. Eur Spine J. 2007; 16(3):431–437

[2] Hasegawa T, Mikawa Y, Watanabe R, An HS. Morphometric analysis of the lumbosacral nerve roots and dorsal root ganglia by magnetic resonance imaging. Spine. 1996; 21(9):1005–1009

[3] Choi KC, Park CK. Percutaneous endoscopic lumbar discectomy for L5-S1 disc herniation: consideration of the relation between the iliac crest and L5-S1 disc. Pain Physician. 2016; 19(2):E301–E308

24 Endoscopic Revision Surgery

Ralf Wagner and Christoph P. Hofstetter

24.1 Principles

Full-endoscopic spine surgery allows for access and revision of previously operated spinal segments. Many surgical principles of traditional surgery also apply to full-endoscopic spine surgery; however, given the small size of the surgical field, it is crucial that principal anatomical landmarks are unambiguously identified. This is even more important for revision surgery where these anatomical landmarks might be obscured by scar tissue or might have been partially resected. Inability to identify principal anatomical landmarks places neural structures at risk as they are typically localized and identified utilizing these landmarks. For interlaminar revision surgeries, the yellow ligament attachment ventral to the rostral lamina is the principal anatomical landmark, since it allows for safe identification of the dura. Alternatively, the medial aspect of the caudal index-level pedicle can serve as an anatomical landmark to localize neural structures. For transforaminal approaches, the caudal pedicle constitutes the principal anatomical landmark. Additional assistance to localize the neural structures may be obtained by using intraoperative electrical stimulation eliciting lower extremity electromyogram (EMG). As with traditional surgery, principal anatomical landmarks should be identified visually and confirmed with the help of fluoroscopy or navigation. This typically allows for safe identification of neural elements, which can be dissected into the scar tissue. The continuous fluid irrigation of full-endoscopic spine surgery is very helpful to dissect scar tissue as it facilitates separation of tissue planes. Moreover, superior high-definition visualization provided by modern endoscopic systems helps us to unambiguously identify landmarks and neural tissue. Finally, the bevel of the tubular retractor is a very helpful component of revision surgery as it serves as a Cobb elevator for developing planes and retraction of neural elements. In conclusion, scarred anatomical planes such as the bone surface or dura are safer identified and dissected in full-endoscopic spine surgery compared to traditional surgery.

24.2 Indications

Decompression of residual/recurrent foraminal, central, or lateral recess stenosis are appropriate indications for full-endoscopic revision surgery. Relative contraindications include vertical foraminal stenosis (foraminal height < 10 mm), segmental coronal deformity with unilateral foraminal collapse, and foraminal stenosis due to scoliotic deformity (coronal Cobb angle > 20 degrees). In these cases, foraminal decompression requires partial resection of the caudal pedicle. While technically feasible, these surgeries are associated with long operative times, potential risk to the exiting nerve root, and typically a short durability of symptomatic relief. For such cases, indirect foraminal decompression via interbody cages with arthrodesis should be considered. Segmental instability due to pars fracture is another relative contraindication to endoscopic revision

surgery. For the revision of arthrodesis constructs, decompression surgeries of neural elements within the successful arthrodesis construct have an excellent outcome. Minimal decompression of neural elements is needed given the lack of mobility and obtained symptomatic relief is typically permanent. Given the advent of powerful high-speed burrs, partial resection of misplaced interbody cages, screws, and other hardware is feasible and can in some cases avoid highly invasive traditional revision surgeries. Decompression of segments adjacent to fusion surgeries is typically less durable given the high biomechanical forces and accelerated degeneration. Central and lateral recess stenosis at adjacent level is often feasible and associated with reasonable durability of symptomatic relief (2–5 years). Foraminal stenosis adjacent to a previous fusion surgery often requires arthrodesis surgery. Dynamic flexion and extension X-rays, CT scans, and MRI are necessary to evaluate adjacent levels prior to any treatment decisions.

24.3 Illustrative Cases

24.3.1 Interlaminar Endoscopic Lumbar Diskectomy Revision

A 40-year-old woman with a past medial history of hypertension, diabetes mellitus, and depression and a surgical history of three previous left L5/S1 diskectomies presents with a 6-month history of pain radiating into her left posterior thigh and calf. The patient describes the pain as stabbing and aching and she rates the pain as 7/10. The patient also complains of 8/10 back pain and was severely disabled (Oswestry Disability Index [ODI]: 68). All conservative means of treatment including NSAIDs (nonsteroidal anti-inflammatory drugs), gabapentin, muscle relaxant, and physical therapy had been attempted. On physical examination, the patient had lower left extremity plantar flexion weakness (3/5) and the left ankle jerk reflex was missing. Preoperative MRI of the L-spine confirmed adequate posterior decompression of the traversing S1 nerve root (▶ Fig. 24.1 **a**). However, the nerve root was severely displaced and impinged by a large ventral disk–osteophyte complex. A CT scan revealed large marginal osteophytes originating from the index-level endplates (▶ Fig. 24.1 **b**). The patient underwent a left L5/S1 interlaminar endoscopic lumbar diskectomy revision with resection of the disk–osteophyte complex. Safe identification of the left S1 nerve root was feasible after additional resection of S1 lamina just medial to the S1 pedicle. Scarred in neural structures were mobilized using the bevel of the tubular retractor (▶ Fig. 24.2 **a**). The disk–osteophyte complex was resected with a diamond burr while retracting the traversing S1 nerve root with tubular retractor (▶ Fig. 24.2 **b**). A postoperative CT scan confirmed complete resection of the disk–osteophyte complex (▶ Fig. 24.2 **c,d**). The patient tolerated the procedure well. She is currently 2 years after the procedure and her strength and sensation have improved. The radicular pain has resolved, and she has minimal residual S1 numbness.

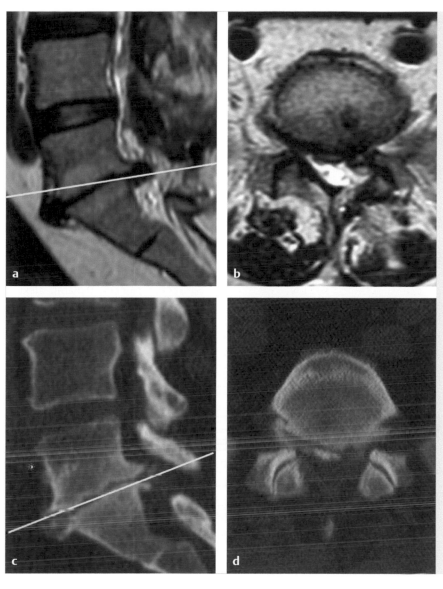

Fig. 24.1 Residual disk–osteophyte complex depicted by preoperative imaging. **(a,b)** Sagittal and axial T2-weighted MRI depict a left L5/S1 disk–osteophyte complex displacing the traversing S1 nerve root posteriorly. Note the extensive posterior decompression on the sagittal image. **(c,d)** A preoperative CT scan reveals large marginal osteophytes originating from the posterior endplates of L5 and S1.

Pearls and Pitfalls

- The caudal index-level pedicle is a useful anatomical landmark in interlaminar approaches for identification of neural elements in severely scarred surgical fields.
- The tubular retractor once advanced into the spinal canal allows for mobilization, retraction, and protection of the neural elements.
- The interlaminar approach allows for resection of disk–osteophyte complexes ventral to the traversing nerve root, in particular in the lower lumbar segments.

24.3.2 Transforaminal Endoscopic Lumbar Diskectomy Revision

A 50-year-old man with a past surgical history of a traditional L4/L5 diskectomy 5 years prior presented with rapid-onset recurrent left lower extremity pain and weakness. The patient described the pain as radiating from his lower back to the

lateral aspect of the thigh and calf and rated it as 7/10 in severity. On neurological examination, the patient had left gluteus medius weakness (4/5). Preoperative imaging revealed a left L4/L5 subarticular disk herniation with minimal downward migration (▶ Fig. 24.3 **a,b**). The patient underwent a left transforaminal endoscopic lumbar L4/L5 diskectomy. Following exposure of the caudal index-level pedicle, the traversing nerve root and the impinging disk fragment were visualized (▶ Fig. 24.3 **c**). The sequester was resected and the annular defect inspected and cleared of loose fragments. Thus, the traversing nerve root was visualized and decompressed spanning from the annulus to the rostral aspect of the pedicle (▶ Fig. 24.3 **d**). The patient tolerated the procedure well and his radiculopathy and weakness have resolved at his 6-month follow-up visit.

Pearls and Pitfalls

- The transforaminal approach provides a virgin surgical corridor for revision diskectomy.

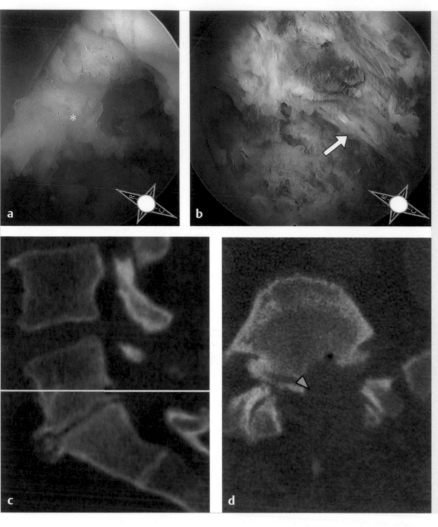

Fig. 24.2 Interlaminar endoscopic lumbar diskectomy revision. **(a)** Intraoperative images reveal a large anterior disk–osteophyte complex. **(b)** The traversing S1 nerve root (*arrow*) reveals epidural scarring but is entirely decompressed ventrally after resection of the disk–osteophyte complex. Postoperative **(c)** sagittal and **(d)** axial CT scan reveals complete resection of the disk–osteophyte complex. The interlaminar approach allowed for resection of the osteophyte–disk complex beyond midline (*green arrowhead*).

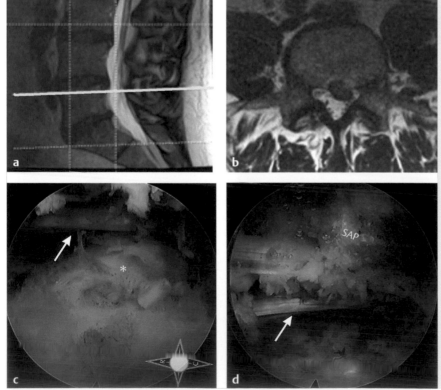

Fig. 24.3 Recurrent left L4/L5 disk herniation. **(a)** Sagittal and **(b)** axial T2-weighted MRI of the lumbar spine depicts a left L4/L5 subarticular disk herniation. **(c)** Intraoperative image depicts the traversing nerve root (*arrow*) displaced by the disk fragment (*asterisk*). **(d)** A complete decompression of the traversing nerve root (*arrow*) is achieved following resection of the fragment. Abbreviation: SAP, superior articular process.

24.3.3 Interlaminar Endoscopic Lateral Recess Decompression Revision

A 71-year-old man with a surgical history of a minimally invasive left L3/L4 medial facetectomy 1 year prior presented with recurrent symptoms. The patient stated that the previous surgery provided relief of his radicular pain but left him with a left foot drop. Three months prior to presentation, he experienced recurrent stabbing pain radiating into the left buttock and lateral thigh, which he rated as 7 out of 10 in severity. The patient states that standing and walking aggravate the pain. On neurological examination, the patient had weakness of his left foot dorsiflexion (0/5), extensor hallucis longus (0/5), and left gluteus medius (3/5). A preoperative lumbar MRI depicts scar tissue in the left L3/L4 lateral recess with scarring and compression of the left traversing L4 nerve root (▶ Fig. 24.4 **a, b**). A preoperative CT scan revealed a postoperative defect in the left L3/L4 facet joint (▶ Fig. 24.4 **c**). He underwent a left L3/L4 interlaminar endoscopic lateral recess decompression. During the procedure, the lateral margin of the neural elements was identified rostral and caudal to the scar tissue of the previous surgery (▶ Fig. 24.4 **d**). The scar tissue was partially resected utilizing a micro-punch. Using an elevator, the scar was dissected off the neural elements (▶ Fig. 24.4 **e**). The scar tissue was densely adherent to the traversing nerve root and therefore left in place (▶ Fig. 24.4 **f**). The traversing nerve root was gently medialized with the bevel of the tubular retractor to rule out any adhesions. The patient tolerated the procedure well. He is currently 6 months after the surgery and his radicular pain has resolved. He did not experience any recovery of his motor strength.

Pearls and Pitfalls

- During the interlaminar approach, the neural elements are safest identified in the rostral surgical field or, alternatively, the traversing nerve root may be identified medial to the caudal index-level pedicle.
- A blunt dissector may be used to dissect neural elements; constant irrigation assists in developing tissue planes.

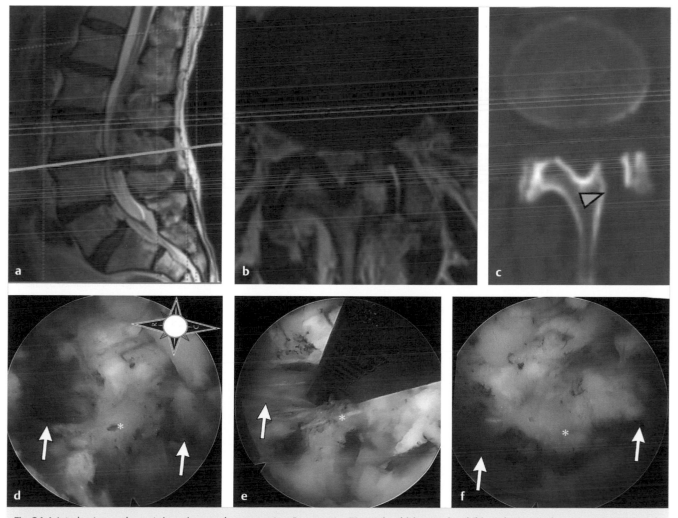

Fig. 24.4 Interlaminar endoscopic lateral recess decompression. Preoperative T2-weighted **(a)** sagittal and **(b)** axial MRI reveals compression of the left L4 nerve root in the left L3/L4 lateral recess. **(c)** Scar tissue is seen in the lateral recess underlying the previous bony decompression. A CT scan depicts the bony defect (*green arrowhead*) of the previous decompression. **(d)** Following the medial facetectomy, the lateral margin of the neural elements (*arrows*) are identified cephalad and caudal to the surgical scar tissue (*asterisk*). **(e)** The nerve root (*arrow*) is gently dissected off the scar tissue (*asterisk*) using a blunt dissector. **(f)** The scar tissue (*asterisk*) is densely adherent to the traversing nerve root (*arrows*) and therefore left in place.

- The interlaminar lateral recess decompression allows for a wide rostrocaudal decompression and for inspection of the neural elements, which is invaluable in the cases of vaguely defined pathology.

24.3.4 Transforaminal Endoscopic Lateral Recess Decompression Revision

A 74-year-old general surgeon with a past surgical history of an L4/L5 laminectomy 5 years prior presented with progressive left lower extremity pain in an L5 distribution. He had minimal weakness in his left extensor hallucis longus (4/5). A diagnostic nerve block confirmed L5 pathology. Preoperative MRI showed left L4/L5 lateral recess stenosis (▶ Fig. 24.5 **a,b**). The patient underwent a left transforaminal endoscopic lateral recess decompression. For the procedure, a trans-superior articular

process (trans-SAP) approach was elected in order to allow for ventral and dorsal decompression of the lateral recess (▶ Fig. 24.5 **c,d**). The ventral SAP was resected using a side-biting burr and a Kerrison rongeur. Resection of the marginal osteophytes was performed using a side-biting burr. The patient tolerated the procedure well. A postoperative CT confirmed adequate decompression of the lateral recess (▶ Fig. 24.5 **e,f**). He is now 6 months after the surgery and his lower extremity radiculopathy has resolved.

Pearls and Pitfalls

- The transforaminal approach utilizing a trans-SAP technique allows for ventral and dorsal decompression of the lateral recess.
- The transforaminal approach provides a virgin surgical corridor for lateral recess decompression revision.

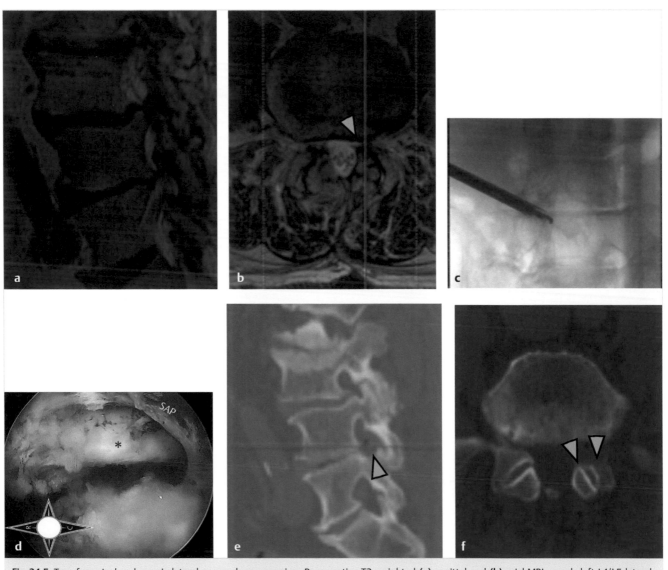

Fig. 24.5 Transforaminal endoscopic lateral recess decompression. Preoperative T2-weighted **(a)** sagittal and **(b)** axial MRI reveals left L4/L5 lateral recess stenosis (*green arrowhead*). Note the missing posterior bony elements s/p previous traditional laminectomy. **(c)** Fluoroscopic verification of the L5 pedicle. **(d)** Intraoperative view of the left L4/L5 lateral recess. The traversing nerve root (*asterisk*) has been decompressed dorsally by resection of the ventral portion of the superior articular process (SAP) and ventrally by resection of marginal osteophytes. Postoperative **(e)** sagittal and **(f)** axial CT reveals adequate decompression of the lateral recess by resection of the ventral aspect of the SAP (*green arrowheads*).

24.3.5 Interlaminar Endoscopic Approach for Resection of Retropulsed Interbody Cage

A 39-year-old woman with a past surgical history of an L4/S1 transforaminal interbody fusion 9 years prior presents with a several year history of progressive right-sided posterolateral thigh and calf pain. On examination, she had right extensor hallucis longus weakness (3/5). Preoperative MRI and CT revealed a posterior displacement of an L5/S1 peek interbody spacer with impingement of the traversing S1 nerve root (▶ Fig. 24.6 **a,b**). The patient underwent an *interlaminar endoscopic partial resection of the interbody cage* for decompression of the right L5/S1 lateral recess. During the operation, the neural elements were identified after minimal additional L5 laminotomy. The bevel of the tubular retractor was utilized to dissect off the scarred neural elements from the posterior aspect of the cage as well as to protect the neural elements during partial resection of the cage (▶ Fig. 24.6 **c**). The patient tolerated the procedure well and experienced complete remission of symptoms. A postoperative CT scan confirmed complete resection of the protruding part of the interbody spacer (▶ Fig. 24.6 **d**).

Pearls and Pitfalls

- Given the small diameter of full-endoscopic technique, pathology within arthrodesis constructs may be accessed in between previously placed instrumentation.
- The tubular retractor allows for mobilization, retraction, and protection of scarred neural elements once advanced into the spinal canal during the interlaminar approach.

24.3.6 Transforaminal Endoscopic Thoracic Diskectomy Revision

A 61-year-old woman with a history of an attempted T12/L1 laminectomy, diskectomy, and fusion (▶ Fig. 24.7 **a**) complicated by a CSF (cerebrospinal fluid) leak treated with 2 weeks of lumbar drainage, and blood patches presented with persistent bilateral thigh and calf cramps. On neurological examination, the patient had right knee extension weakness (4/5) and was myelopathic (left positive Babinski's sign). Preoperative MRI depicted a large central T12/L1 disk protrusion with impingement of the spinal cord (▶ Fig. 24.7 **b**). The patient underwent a left T12/L1 transforaminal endoscopic thoracic diskectomy. During the procedure, an approximately 4×2 mm large defect of the ventrolateral thecal sac was seen, which was reconstructed using a DuraGen inlay graft and TISSEEL (▶ Fig. 24.7 **c e**). The patient tolerated the procedure well and a postoperative MRI confirmed complete resection of the disk herniation (▶ Fig. 24.7 **f**). Twelve months after her full-endoscopic revision surgery, her lower extremity cramps have resolved.

Pearls and Pitfalls

- The transforaminal approach allows for access to pathology ventral to the thoracic spinal cord.
- Full-endoscopic spine surgery may in certain cases avoid complications associated with traditional surgery.

24.3.7 Interlaminar Endoscopic Approach for Resection of Sacroiliac Bolt

A 56-year old female patient with a history of an L2/L5 fusion developed acute right S1 radiculopathy following a right

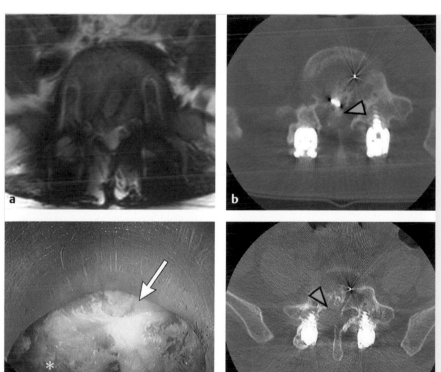

Fig. 24.6 Interlaminar endoscopic resection of intervertebral spacer. Preoperative (a) axial MRI and (b) CT depicts lateral recess stenosis by a protruding spacer. (c) Intraoperative view of the medial aspect of the spacer following partial resection. (d) Postoperative CT confirms adequate decompression.

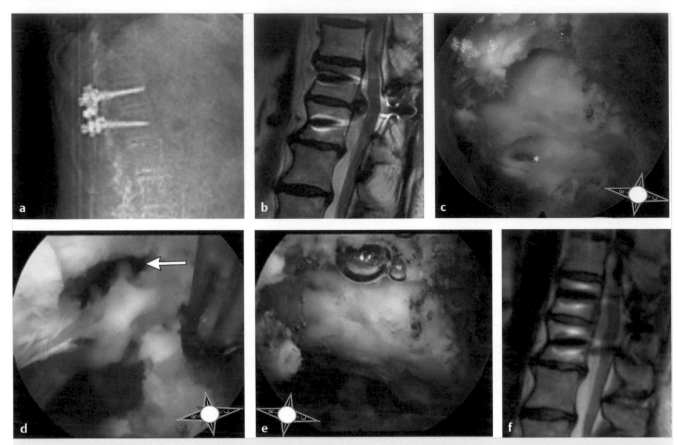

Fig. 24.7 Transforaminal endoscopic thoracic diskectomy. **(a)** Preoperative X-ray depicts a T12/L1 pedicle screw–rod construct. **(b)** Preoperative T2-weighed MRI shows a central T12/L1 disk herniation with impingement of the thoracic spinal cord. **(c)** Intraoperative image of the disk herniation (*asterisk*) impinging the spinal cord. **(d)** The dural defect (*arrow*) from the index surgery is inspected. **(e)** Upon resection of the disk herniation, the spinal cord is decompressed. **(f)** A postoperative MRI confirms adequate decompression of the spinal cord.

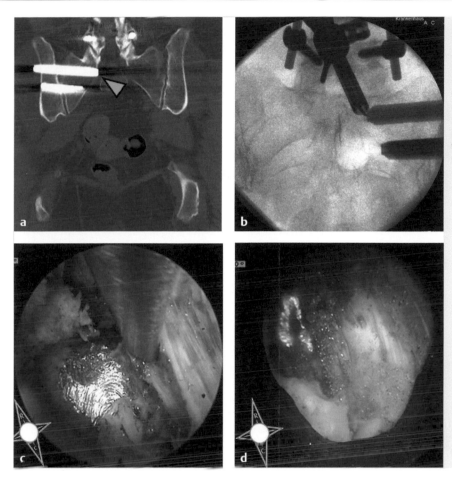

Fig. 24.8 Interlaminar endoscopic partial resection of sacroiliac (SI) bolt. **(a)** Preoperative coronal CT reveals protruding of the cephalad SI bolt beyond the medial surface of the S1 pedicle (*arrowhead*). **(b)** Intraoperative anteroposterior fluoroscopic image confirms appropriate position of the endoscope. **(c)** Retraction of the traversing S1 nerve root exposes the tip of the SI bolt. **(d)** After partial resection of the SI bolt, no further compression of the traversing nerve root is noted.

sacroiliac fusion. The patient described sharp pain radiating into her right posterior calf. She was intact on neurological examination. Preoperative CT revealed that the superior sacroiliac bolt protruded beyond the S1 *pedicle* (▶ Fig. 24.8 **a**). The patient underwent an interlaminar endoscopic right hemilaminotomy for resection of the protruding sacroiliac bolt (▶ Fig. 24.8 **b**). Intraoperatively, the tip of the SI bolt was noted to displace the S1 nerve root (▶ Fig. 24.8 **c**). Using a diamond burr, the protruding part of the sacroiliac bolt was resected (▶ Fig. 24.8 **d**). The patient tolerated the procedure well and her radicular pain resolved.

Pearls and Pitfalls

- Small protruding parts of titanium instrumentation may be resected using endoscopic diamond burrs.

25 Complications Associated with Full-Endoscopic Spine Surgery

Jun Ho Lee and Christoph P. Hofstetter

25.1 Types of Complications

Analysis of traditional spine surgery has shown that surgical invasiveness is strongly associated with the rate of complications in multiple organ systems.[1] The rationale of minimally invasive spine surgery and in particular full-endoscopic spine surgery is to decrease the invasiveness and thus the rate of systemic and surgical complications. The following complications have been reported following full-endoscopic spine surgery: durotomies, epidural hematomas, postoperative paresthesias, incomplete resection of disk herniations, complex regional pain syndrome, and systemic complications.[2] Infections may occur but appear to be exceedingly rare given that the instruments do not have any direct contact with the skin and that surgeries are performed under continuous irrigation (▶ Table 25.1).

25.2 Dural Lacerations

Several features of full-endoscopic spine surgery help avoid dural lacerations. The high-definition off-axis visualization allows direct visualization of every aspect of tissue resection when using Kerrison rongeurs, micro-punches, or burrs (for surgical technique, see Chapters 8 and 9). Moreover, continuous irrigation decreases the transmural pressure gradient of the thecal sac and allows for easier and safer manipulation of neural structures. However, dural lacerations can occur during any endoscopic approach, and the spine surgeon performing these type of surgeries needs to be familiar with appropriate management strategies.[3]

25.2.1 Dural Lacerations Encountered during the Transforaminal Approach

When performing a transforaminal approach, the highest risk of dural laceration is during the initial in-line dissection. Both the nonvisualized (utilizing bone reamers) and visualized (resecting disk/posterior longitudinal ligament) expose the neural elements to potential damage. The following conditions increase the risk of dural laceration during transforaminal cases:
- Previous interlaminar surgery (traversing nerve root is adherent).
- Utilization of bone reamers in the upper lumbar segments (L1/L2 and L2/L3).
- Traversing nerve root is deviated laterally by a subarticular disk herniation.
- Revision transforaminal surgery.
- Extensive foraminal osteophytes.
- Calcified thoracic disks.

The risk of damage to the exiting nerve root is minimized by careful preoperative analysis of the foraminal size and the location of the exiting nerve root in the foramen. In the cases of severe foraminal stenosis or an inferior location of the nerve root, a trans-superior articular process (trans-SAP)/extraforaminal approach should be considered. Damage to the traversing nerve root with the bone reamer can be avoided by respecting the medial pedicle line on anteroposterior (AP) fluoroscopic imaging during SAP resection. Of note, in the upper lumbar spine (L1/L2 and L2/L3), the thecal sac may extend beyond the medial pedicle line and therefore bone reaming should be carried out only to the mid-portion of the pedicle on AP fluoroscopic imaging. Nerve root damage during resection of the disk/posterior longitudinal ligament can be avoided by first identifying the traversing nerve root at the medial aspect of the caudal index-level pedicle and then carefully dissecting off the nerve root from the disk pathology. In the cases with scarring or severe pathology, intraoperative electrophysiological mapping helps identify and protect neural structures.

25.2.2 Case Examples

A 59-year-old man presented with right L4 radicular pain that he rates as 9/10 in severity. The patient experienced complete transient relief by a diagnostic block. Preoperative MRI confirmed right L4/L5 foraminal stenosis (▶ Fig. 25.1 **a**). The patient underwent a right L4/L5 transforaminal endoscopic lumbar foraminotomy (TELF) using the trans-SAP technique. Bone trephines were utilized for partial resection of the right L5 SAP. Upon insertion of the endoscope, a laceration of the traversing nerve root sleeve caused by bony reamer was noted (▶ Fig. 25.1 **b**). The arachnoid appeared to be intact and the traversing nerve root was seen. No frank bulging or herniation of the nerve root was noted. The foraminotomy was completed and the operative field was filled with TISSEEL. Six months after surgery, the patient's constant leg pain has resolved. However, he experiences episodes of sharp pain with physical exertion such as heavy lifting.

A 58-year-old man presents with rapid-onset burning anterior thigh pain, which he rates as 9/10 in severity. On examination, the patient has right hip flexor weakness (3/5).

Table 25.1 Multicenter cohort study of patients treated by surgeons within Endoscopic Spine Study Group (553 endoscopic surgeries)

Complications	Rate
Durotomy	4 (0.72%)
Epidural hematoma	2 (0.36%)
Complex pain disorder	2 (0.36%)
Recurrent disk herniation	4 (1.1%)
Persistent disk herniation	10 (1.8%)
Systemic	4 (1.8%)
Total	2 (4.7%)

Note: The cohort's mean age was 57 years. The following pathologies were treated:
- Disk herniations (377, 68%).
- Central stenosis (71, 12%).
- Foraminal stenosis (68, 12%).
- Other pathologies: lateral recess stenosis, adjacent segment disease, synovial cysts, and diskitis (8%).

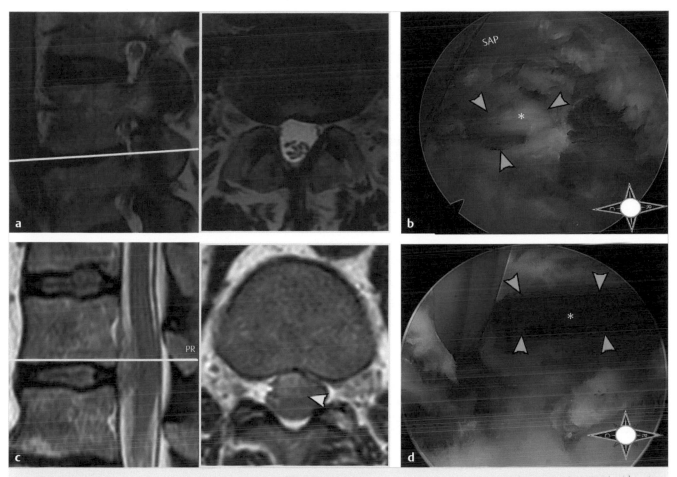

Fig. 25.1 Dural lacerations during transforaminal approaches. (a) MRI depicts preoperative sagittal and axial T2 weighted MRI of a patient with L4/L5 foraminal stenosis. (b) Intraoperative image of a dural laceration (*asterisk*) caused by the initial reaming (*green arrowheads*, edges of the dura; *asterisk*, dura, SAP, superior articular process). (c) Preoperative thoracic T2-weighted MRI depicts intradural disk herniation at T11/T12 with displacement of the spinal cord. *Yellow arrowhead* depicts the intradural disk fragment. (d) Intraoperative view of the ventral dural defect. *Green arrowheads* indicate the edges of the ventral dural defect (*asterisk*).

Preoperative MRI reveals a T11/T12 disk herniation with efface-ment of the CSF space and displacement of the spinal cord (▶ Fig. 25.1 c). High-resolution T2 images suggest an intradural location of the fragment. The patient underwent a right T11/T12 transforaminal endoscopic thoracic diskectomy (TETD). Upon partial resection of the T12 SAP, the neural structures were iden-tified and dissected off the disk material located ventrally to the thecal sac. Once the disk sequester was retrieved, a ventral dural defect was noted (▶ Fig. 25.1 **d**). An inlay DuraGen graft was placed and secured in place with TISSEEL. Six months after his surgery, the patient is off all pain medications and his right thigh pain has resolved. His neurological examination has normalized.

25.2.3 Dural Lacerations Encountered during the Interlaminar Approach

When performing an interlaminar approach, the highest risk of dural laceration is during transgression of the yellow ligament. Conditions that increase the risk of accidental laceration of the dura include the following:
- Extremely severe stenosis.
- Stenosis with associated spondylolisthesis or scoliosis.
- Previous lumbar epidural steroid injections.
- Previous surgery.
- Synovial cysts.
- Old age.
- Smoking.

If the yellow ligament is thinned out or transgressed during the bony decompression, that opening should be used for resection of the yellow ligament utilizing off-axis resection technique (see Chapter 9 for details regarding off-axis technique). If in-line dissection of the yellow ligament is necessary, it is best accomplished in a paramedian plane. Transgressing the yellow ligament too far off-midline may result in exposure lateral to the neural elements, which is most likely to occur at L5/S1. In the median plane along the midline raphe, the yellow ligament/epidural fat/dura planes can sometimes be difficult to discern. In-line dissection of the yellow ligament is best accomplished using a micro-punch (see Chapter 9 for details regarding in-line technique). Alternatively, it may be transgressed with a blunt dissector or Kerrison rongeur. Identification of neural elements can be facilitated by resecting more lamina rostrally or caudally. During the latter, the medial aspect of the caudal index-level pedicle constitutes as reliable bony landmark for safe identifica-tion of the neural elements.

25.2.4 Case Examples

A 68-year-old woman presented with past surgical history of L4/S1 fusion and status post-L3/L4 endoscopic unilateral laminotomy for bilateral decompression (ULBD) for adjacent-level degeneration 3 years prior to presentation. The patient complained of pain radiating into her left anterior thigh and was neurologically intact. Preoperative imaging revealed an L3/L4 degenerative segmental coronal deformity with left vertical foraminal stenosis and a left synovial cyst (▶ Fig. 25.2 **a**). The patient underwent an extreme lateral interbody fusion with a lateral plate and a revision ULBD with resection of the synovial cyst. During the attempted transgression of the yellow ligament at the inferior edge of the L3 lamina, the scarred dura was

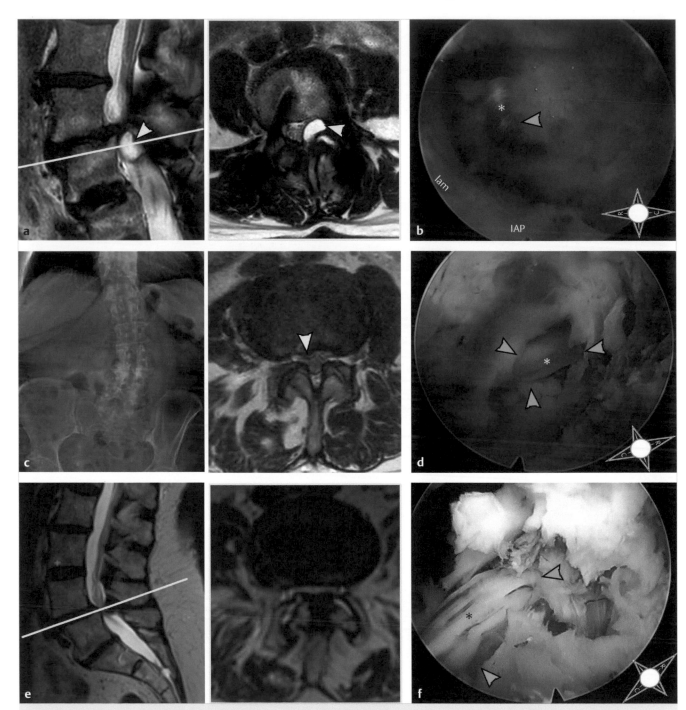

Fig. 25.2 Dural lacerations during interlaminar approaches. **(a)** Sagittal and axial T2-weighted MR images of the lumbar spine reveal a left L3/L4 synovial cyst causing impingement of the neural elements (*yellow arrowheads*). **(b)** Intraoperative view depicts a small laceration of the dura (*asterisk*) with herniation of nerve roots (*green arrowhead*). **(c)** Patient with lumbar levoscoliosis and severe right L4/L5 lateral recess stenosis (*yellow arrowhead*). **(d)** Intraoperative image depicts a dural defect (*green arrowheads*) in the lateral recess. Note the thinning of the thecal sac medial to the defect. **(e)** Sagittal and axial T2-weighted MR images depict high-grade L4/L5 stenosis with a grade 1 anterolisthesis. **(f)** Intraoperative view depicts a wide central dural defect. The edge of the remaining dura is ill defined (*green arrowheads*). Abbreviations: IAP, inferior articular process; lam, lamina.

mistaken for yellow ligament. Using a blunt dissector, a small opening of the dura was produced, and nerve roots were noted to herniate through the defect (▶ Fig. 25.2 **b**). The ULBD and resection of the synovial cyst were completed. Prior to closure, the dural defect was repaired with a DuraGen inlay graft and sealed with TISSEEL. The patient is 3 months after surgery and her symptoms have resolved.

A 65-year-old woman presents with right flank pain and pain radiating into her right anterolateral thigh. On examination, the patient had right dorsiflexion weakness (4/5). Preoperative scoliosis X-rays reveal 20 degrees of lumbar levoscoliosis and a lumbar MRI confirms right L3/L4 and L4/L5 lateral recess stenosis (▶ Fig. 25.2 **c**). The patient underwent a right L3/L4 and L4/L5 interlaminar endoscopic lateral recess decompression. During the L4/L5 decompression, thinning of the dura was noted close to the midline. Utilizing carefully off-axis resection of the highly stenotic lamina and facet joint, a dural defect was detected in the lateral aspect of the thecal sac within the lateral recess (▶ Fig. 25.2 **d**). The lateral recess decompression was completed and the dural defect was repaired with a DuraGen inlay graft secured with TISSEEL.

A 75-year-old woman presents with neurogenic claudication due to severe L4/L5 spinal stenosis with grade 1 anterolisthesis (▶ Fig. 25.2 **e**). The patients underwent an L4/5 endoscopic ULBD. During in-line transgression of the yellow ligament arachnoid was encountered. Utilizing careful off-axis dissection the frail edges of the dural lining were detected (▶ Fig. 25.2 **f**). The decompression was completed and the large central dural defect was covered with a DuraGen onlay graft. TISSEEL was applied to keep the DuraGen in place. Six months after the procedure, the patient has residual 4/10 buttock pain with ambulation or riding the bicycle. The patient is treated conservatively with COX-1 (cyclooxygenase-1) inhibitors (Cerebrex).

25.3 Dural Lacerations in Full-Endoscopic Spine Surgery

25.3.1 Clinical Symptoms

In contrast to traditional surgery, frank cerebrospinal fluid leaks through the skin are exceptionally rare in full-endoscopic spine surgery. This is due to the lack of dead space along the surgical corridor serving as a conduit for cerebrospinal fluid in traditional surgery. Patients typically become symptomatic when nerve roots herniate out of the thecal sac. Thus, dural defects in the cervical and thoracic are commonly asymptomatic. In the lumbar spine, lateral dural lacerations may cause radicular symptoms with exertion or Valsalva maneuvers. In case of large central lacerations during ULBD, the patient may encounter sacral midline pain with physical activity and with change of body position.

25.3.2 Management Algorithm

Avoidance is the best management strategy for dural lacerations. However, once a dural defect has occurred, the following algorithm has been utilized:
- Small dural defect with intact arachnoid and no herniation of nerve roots:
  - TISSEEL applied with two 18-G needles via the working channel.

- Small dural defect with herniation of nerve roots:
  - DuraGen inlay graft secured with TISSEEL.
- Large dural defect with herniation of nerve roots:
  - DuraGen onlay graft secured with TISSEEL.
  - *Alternatively*, conversion to open surgery for traditional dural repair.

Patients at risk of nerve root herniation are typically kept flat for 24 hours after surgery and then mobilized.

25.3.3 Surgical Technique

Even after a dural laceration has occurred, completion of surgical objectives should be attempted if safely possible. Frank herniation of cauda equina rootlets into the surgical field and the working channel may hinder this endeavor. Utilizing the bevel of the working sleeve to contain nerve roots may be attempted but should be carried out cautiously in order to avoid injury to the rootlets. For surgical repair of a medium size dural defect, an inlay graft is brought in rolled up utilizing cup forceps (▶ Fig. 25.3 **a,b**). We typically use DuraGen, but other materials such as Alloderm may be used. The intended inlay graft should be sized a bit larger in its diameter compared to the dural defect and should cover every corner of lacerated perimeter (a coverage in subdural fashion). Using either forceps or a nerve hook, the inlay graft is carefully tucked under the edges of the dural defect (▶ Fig. 25.3 **c**). Insertion of the inlay graft may be tedious given the inability of true bimanual surgical manipulation in full-endoscopic spine surgery. The bevel of the tubular retractor or a slightly bent K-wire brought in via an irrigation channel allows us to secure areas of the inlay graft that are in appropriate position, while the remaining parts of the inlay graft are tucked under the edge of the dural defect (▶ Fig. 25.3 **d,e**). Moreover, rigorous control of the irrigation fluid can be helpful to achieve optimal placement of the inlay graft. Once the graft is in place, two 18-G needles are advanced into the working channel and fibrin glue is carefully infused to secure the graft in place (▶ Fig. 25.3 **f**).

25.3.4 Pearls and Pitfalls

- Off-axis resection of soft tissue is always safer than in-line resection and should be utilized if possible.
- Early recognition of a dural defect helps avoid additional resection of the thecal sac and significantly alleviates repair.
- Small to medium size dural defects repaired with inlay grafts typically do not affect patient outcome.
- Large dural defects are only partially treated with onlay grafts—in some cases, conversion to traditional surgery may be necessary. Further development of full-endoscopic dural closure techniques is needed.

25.4 Hematomas

As with any other spine surgery, postoperative epidural hematomas can occur following full-endoscopic spine surgery. Symptomatic epidural hematomas typically lead to back pain and radicular motor deficits corresponding to the site of surgery. The timing and presentation are similar to traditional spine surgery. Thrombocytopenia, coagulation disorders, or

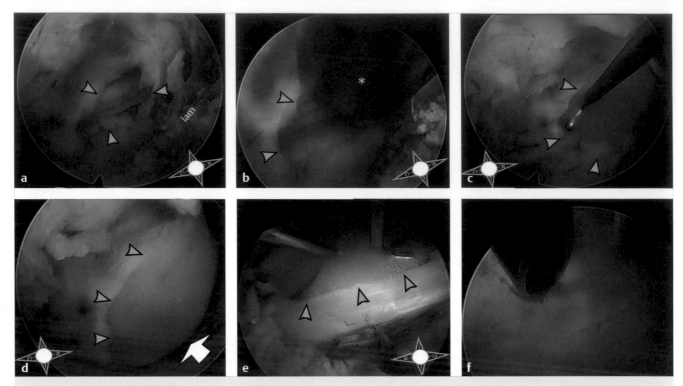

Fig. 25.3 Dural tear repair technique. **(a)** A laceration of the thecal sac is noted in the lateral recess during an interlaminar endoscopic lateral recess decompression. The dural edges are demarked by green arrowheads in **(a–e)**. **(b)** A DuraGen inlay graft (*asterisk*) is brought in with cup forceps. **(c)** Utilizing a nerve hook, the inlay graft is tucked under the dural edges. **(d)** During placement, the inlay graft it is partially secured with the bevel of the tubular retractor (*white arrow*) or **(e)** alternatively with a slightly bent K-wire brought in via an irrigation port. **(f)** Two spinal needles are brought in to deliver TISSEEL to secure the repair. Abbreviation: lam, lamina.

pharmaceutical anticoagulation increase intraoperative oozing and the risk of postoperative hematomas. It is possible to leave wound drains following full-endoscopic surgeries if the surgical field hemostasis is insufficient or if the patient requires acute anti-coagulation. Surgical areas prone to bleeding are the following:

- Dorsal to the mid part of the lamina:
  - Interlaminar lumbar approach—typically occurs with a rostral deviation of the approach trajectory while attempting to identify the inferomedial lamina edge.
- Small arterial bone bleeders adjacent to facet joints:
  - ULBD in cases with severe joint degeneration.
- Epidural bleeders under the edge of the laminotomy—typically caused by bites with the Kerrison rongeurs:
  - ULBD.
- Epidural bleeders under the edge of the lateral recess:
  - ULBD.
  - Interlaminar endoscopic lateral recess decompression (IE-LRD).
- Perineural arterioles:
  - Interlaminar contralateral endoscopic lumbar foraminotomy (ICELF).
  - TELF.
- Epidural venous plexus ventral to the thecal sac near the midline:
  - TELF.
  - Transforaminal endoscopic lumbar diskectomy (TELD).
- Facet joint vessels at the lateral aspect of the SAP resection:
  - TELF.
  - TELD.

25.4.1 Case Examples

A 34-year-old male with a past surgical history of a right L5/S1 diskectomy presents with low back pain and right lower extremity pain (8/10). An EMG (electromyogram) confirms right L5 and S1 radiculopathy. A preoperative MRI of the lumbar spine depicts severe foraminal stenosis due to loss of foraminal height and subluxation of the SAP (▶ Fig. 25.4 **a**). The patient underwent a right L5/S1 ICELF (▶ Fig. 25.4 **b**). The procedure was uneventful, and the patient was discharged 2 hours following the procedure. He woke up the morning after the procedure with recurrent leg pain and plantar flexion weakness (4/5). Imaging of the lumbar spine revealed a postoperative epidural hematoma (▶ Fig. 25.4 **c**). He underwent a full-endoscopic wound hema-toma evacuation. Intraoperatively, an actively bleeding perineural arteriole was identified (▶ Fig. 25.4 **d**). Following the evacuation, the patient's neurological deficits resolved.

25.4.2 Pearls and Pitfalls

- Dissection in areas of frequent hemorrhage should be carried out cautiously. Evulsion of perineural arterioles of the exiting nerve roots should be avoided.
- Meticulous hemostasis should be obtained through all stages of the surgery (see Chapter 8).
- Meticulous hemostasis should be confirmed at the end of the procedure with a patent egress port.
- If hemostasis is suboptimal at the end of the procedure a small wound drain may be left in place. In particular for procedures with extensive tissue dissection such as LE-ULBDs.

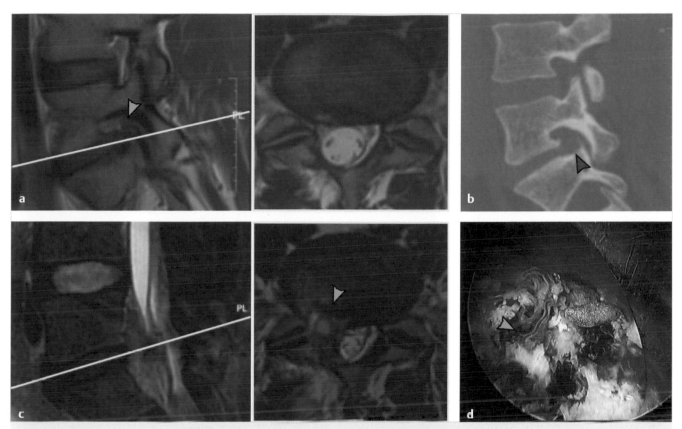

Fig. 25.4 Postoperative hematoma. (a) Preoperative T2-weighted MRI depicts severe foraminal stenosis due to subluxation of the superior articular process (SAP; green arrowhead). (b) Postoperative CT scan confirms resection of the SAP (red arrowhead). (c) MRI depicts a postoperative epidural hematoma (green arrowhead). (d) Intraoperative view of an actively bleeding perineural arteriole (green arrowhead).

25.5 Paresthesias

Postoperative paresthesias are commonly experienced following nerve decompression via interlaminar or transforaminal technique. Symptoms are typically localized in the distribution of the decompressed nerve root and described as tingling/aching sensation. Often patients describe soreness of the innervated muscle groups. Normally, the discomfort is transient and rarely lasts more than 4 to 6 weeks. Two full-endoscopic surgeries are more prone to severe postoperative paresthesias. First, posterior endoscopic cervical foraminotomies, particularly if the nerve root is retracted for resection of ventral osteophytes. In particular, posterior endoscopic cervical foraminotomies in the setting of dense foraminal scarring following high-energy trauma may cause severe postoperative paresthesias with only minimal manipulation. TELF is the other procedure that can lead to severe postoperative paresthesias. High-grade foraminal stenosis or location of the exiting nerve root within the inferior aspect of the foramen increases the risk for postoperative paresthesias. Moreover, a TELF for the L5/S1 foramen is more prone to postoperative paresthesias given the higher nerve-to-foraminal areal ratio, the width of the foramen, and the iliac crest. Utilizing a trans-SAP or extraforaminal approach may help minimize the risk of nerve root irritation. Moreover, performing the surgery in an away patient and limiting the time of intraforaminal work may further decrease the risk. However, alternative direct decompressive procedures such as ICELF or indirect decompression such as anterior lumbar interbody fusion or transforaminal lumbar interbody fusion should be considered.

25.5.1 Case Example

A 54-year-old woman with fibromyalgia and a past surgical history of L3/L4 and L4/L5 laminectomies presents with back pain and right lower extremity pain (9/10) in an L5 radicular distribution. Preoperative imaging revealed vertical foraminal stenosis with a broad-based foraminal disk bulge (▶ Fig. 25.5 a). She underwent right L4/L5 and L5/S1 TELF (▶ Fig. 25.5 b). A postoperative MRI confirmed resection of the bulging foraminal disk (▶ Fig. 25.5 c). Three months after the surgery, the patients complained about 8/10 burning, shooting, and stabbing pain along an L5 distribution. The patient was treated with NSAIDs (nonsteroidal anti-inflammatory drugs), oral steroids, and epidural steroid injection, which alleviated her symptoms.

25.6 Incomplete Transforaminal Endoscopic Lumbar Diskectomy

Transforaminal technique based on the index-level disk as the principal anatomical landmark such as intradiskal or half-in/half-out techniques are associated with the risk of incomplete disk resection.[4] While adjuncts such as labeling of the disk with

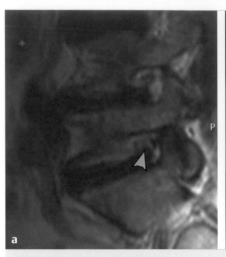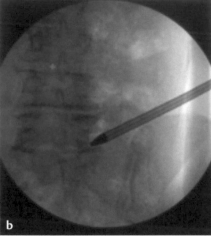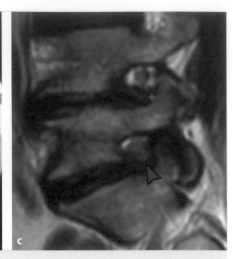

Fig. 25.5 (a) Preoperative MRI reveals an L5/S1 foraminal disk bulge (*green arrowhead*) with compression of the exiting nerve root. **(b)** Rostrocaudal trajectory of the transforaminal endoscopic lumbar foraminotomy. **(c)** Postoperative MRI depicting the resected disk bulge (*red arrowhead*).

indigo carmine dye and frequent fluoroscopic imaging can help with orientation, the soft disk of the index level constitutes no reliable principal anatomical landmark for several reasons:

- The disk cannot be visualized with intraoperative fluoroscopic imaging, which hampers the transition from radiographic localization and palpation to visualization.
- The disk is commonly the site of pathology and therefore often deformed.
- The disk has no well-defined relation to the neural elements as they can be found posterior, lateral, or medial to a protruding fragment.
- Targeting and docking the working sleeve into the disk space result in the creation of a working area ventral to the posterior spinal line/spinal canal. Thus, it does not allow for compete visualization of the neural elements within the spinal canal. During the last decade, several techniques have been developed to achieve partial resection of the ventral SAP (foraminoplasty) to gain access to the medial portion of the caudal index-level pedicle, which is a well-established principal anatomical landmark for spine surgery and allows for straightforward identification of the traversing nerve root. Visualization and identification of the neural elements that are decompressed allows for visual confirmation of complete decompression.

25.6.1 Case Example

A 36-year-old man with a surgical history of a traditional left L4/L5 diskectomy presents with recurrent left lower extremity pain and extensor hallucis longus weakness (4/5). Preoperative imaging reveals that the patient suffered from a recurrent L4/L5 disk herniation with caudal migration (▶ Fig. 25.6 **a–c**). The patient underwent an L4/L5 TELD utilizing half-in/half-out technique without foraminoplasty (▶ Fig. 25.6 **d–f**). Several large disk fragments were retrieved, and pulsations of the epidural fat were noted at the end of the procedure. Postoperatively, the patient experienced persistent left lower extremity pain and weakness. A repeat MRI revealed a retained distal disk fragment (▶ Fig. 25.6 **e–g**). The patient underwent a repeat TELD performing a foraminoplasty and appropriate positioning of the tubular retractor, dorsal to the posterior spinal line (▶ Fig. 25.6 **h,i**). This technique allowed for direct visualization of the neural elements and the retained disk fragment. The fragment was retrieved using grasping forceps and complete decompression of the traversing nerve root was achieved (▶ Fig. 25.7). The patient tolerated the procedure well and experienced complete resolution of his symptoms.

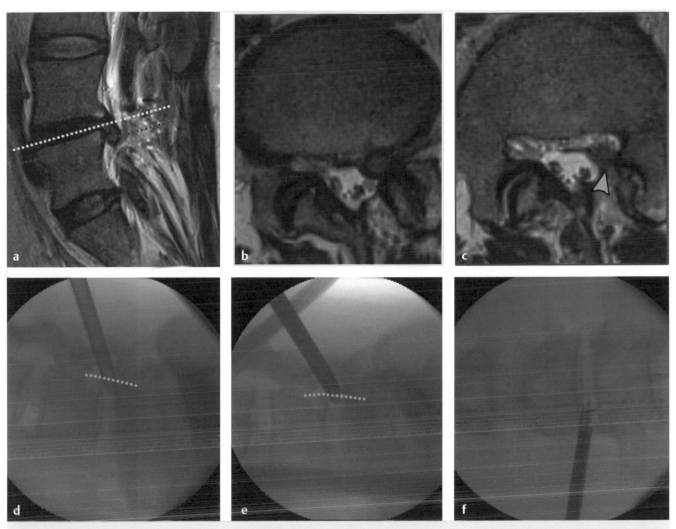

Fig. 25.6 Retained migrated fragment following transforaminal endoscopic lumbar diskectomy. **(a–c)** Preoperative sagittal and axial T2-weighted MRI depicts a left L4/L5 disk herniation with caudal migration. **(d,e)** Intraoperative fluoroscopic images of the index procedure. Note the half-in/half-out position of the bevel of the endoscope. **(f)** Moreover, the grasping forces remain within the confinements of the disk space. (*Continued*)

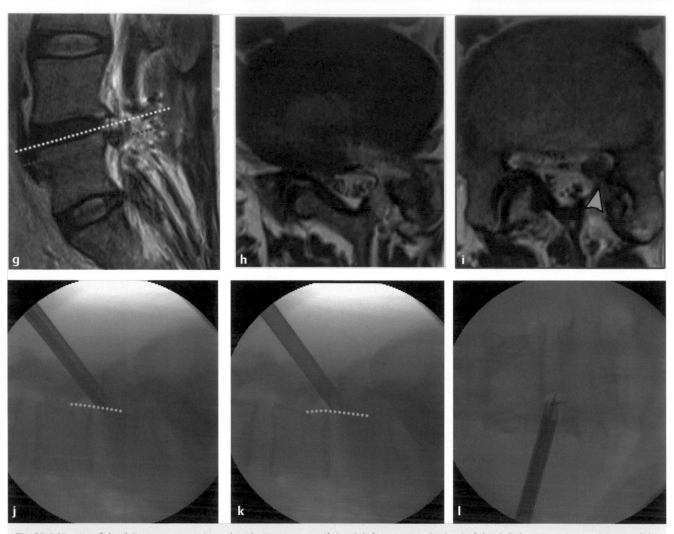

Fig. 25.6 (*Continued*) **(g–i)** Postoperative MRI studies depict resection of the disk fragment at the level of the disk; however, the caudal part of the fragment remains within the lateral recess (*green arrowhead*). **(j,k)** Intraoperative fluoroscopic images of the revision transforaminal endoscopic lumbar diskectomy. Note that the bevel of the tubular retractor remains posterior to the posterior spinal line. **(l)** Moreover, the grasping forceps reach beyond the disk space.

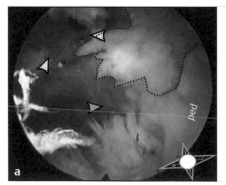

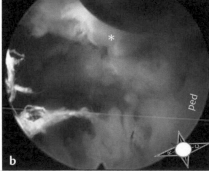

Fig. 25.7 Intraoperative images of transforaminal endoscopic L4/L5 diskectomy revision. **(a)** The green arrowhead points toward the superior endplate of L5. The annular defect of the previous surgery performed utilizing half-in/half-out technique is seen. The rostral portion of the disk fragment is detected (*black dotted line*). Epidural fat (*yellow arrowheads*) is medial to the fragment. **(b)** The disk fragment (*asterisk*) is retrieved with grasping forceps. Abbreviation: ped, pedicle.

25.6.2 Pearls and Pitfalls

- Disk-based targeting for TELD is associated with the risk of incomplete visualization of neural elements and thus incomplete decompression.

- Performing an adequate foraminoplasty allows access to the medial aspect of the caudal index-level pedicle, which serves as the *principal anatomical landmark* for safe localization and direct visualization of neural elements.

26 Perioperative Care in Full-Endoscopic Spine Surgery

Lynn McGrath and Christoph P. Hofstetter

26.1 Introduction

One of the major advantages of full-endoscopic spine surgery is the reduction in surgical site pain, length of hospital stay, and recovery time when compared to minimally invasive surgical (MIS) and traditional open spine surgical techniques. However, understanding and implementation of sound perioperative care is a key factor to ensure that each patient derives the full benefit of full-endoscopic spine surgery. While many of the best practices utilized for perioperative care in the MIS and open surgical patient populations are appropriate for the endoscopic spine surgery population, there are some specific considerations in this cohort that are worth discussing.

26.2 Infection Control

Surgical invasiveness is the most reliable indicator of a surgical site infection after spine surgery.[1] Accordingly, the minimal degree of tissue disruption and destruction afforded by full-endoscopic spine surgery is certainly beneficial in ensuring an extremely low rate of postoperative surgical site infections. The preservation of local vasculature helps the body maintain normal immunological access to the surgical site. Additionally, the near absence of dead space maximizes normal tissue apposition, which optimizes wound healing and limits the potential for the accumulation of fluid or infectious organisms. Other well-validated predictors of postoperative surgical site infection in spine surgery include morbid obesity, hypertension, renal disease, diabetes, and advanced age.[1] Appropriate preoperative medical, metabolic, and nutritional optimization should be considered a vital component to mitigating rates of surgical site infection in any surgical population including those undergoing full-endoscopic spine surgery.

Finally, we recommend following the North American Spine Society's (NASS) Evidence-Based Clinical Guideline on Antibiotic Prophylaxis in Spine Surgery, which suggests, for a typical uncomplicated lumbar laminotomy or diskectomy, a single preoperative dose of antibiotics with intraoperative re-dosing as needed to decrease the risk of infection and/or diskitis.[2]

26.3 Pain Management

Postoperative pain is an inevitable consequence of any surgical technique, with up to 81% of spine patients reporting moderate to severe pain in the postoperative period even after discharge.[3] Thus, despite the minimally invasive nature of endoscopic spine surgery, appropriate pain management is a key principle in ensuring optimal patient recovery, rates of return to work, and patient satisfaction.

While no universally accepted protocol for postoperative pain management has been accepted, there are certain tenets that have been shown to reliably manage pain, minimize hospital length of stay, and lead to improved patient quality of life. Multimodal analgesia is an important principle by which to construct a pain regimen that addresses the problem in a logical and stepwise fashion and begins before the incision is made. While the evidence is not yet definitive, preemptive analgesia with nonsteroidal anti-inflammatory drugs (NSAIDs), cyclooxygenase-2 (COX-2) inhibitors, or anticonvulsants has shown promise in improving health-related quality of life for spine patients.[4] As such, our protocol includes preoperative administration of 1,000 mg of acetaminophen and 1,200 mg of gabapentin in addition to local anesthesia with bupivacaine. Prior to incision, we administer a 0.5 kg/mg ketamine bolus and taper off 30 minutes before the end of surgery. We also administer 30 mg of ketorolac when appropriate, as this has been shown to help achieve optimal postoperative pain control.[5]

Postoperatively, we attempt to limit the use of opioids to episodes of breakthrough pain; consequently, acetaminophen, NSAIDs, and COX-2 inhibitors form the foundation of our postoperative pain regimen. Use of these agents has been shown to reduce opioid requirements by 20 to 30%.[6] In the case of postoperative pain exacerbation or a delay in resolution of preoperative radiculopathy, we find that NSAIDs and steroids in combination with gabapentin often lead to satisfactory symptomatic relief. In the cases where radicular pain is persistent despite optimal medical management, referral for epidural steroid injection may be appropriate.

Full-endoscopic spine surgery nearly always require the passage of the endoscope through a significant amount of muscle tissue, which can lead to muscle spasm and an exacerbation of overall postoperative pain levels with the potential to prolong hospitalization. As such, we find the use of muscle relaxants, especially in young males, to be particularly helpful in minimizing the dose and duration of opioid use. Nonmedical interventions such as early mobilization, thermotherapy, massage, or ultrasound may be helpful for persistent cases.

Regardless of the pain regimen selected, the physician must first be familiar with the side effect profiles of any medication administered and the subsequent use of these medications needs to be informed by the baseline comorbidities and sensitivities of each patient.

26.4 Wound Healing

While it should not be the primary indication for choosing an endoscopic approach, the minimally invasive nature of the full-endoscopic technique does convey to patients the reasonable expectation for an impeccable cosmetic result. Wound management should begin prior to incision. While a small incision is desirable, the surgeon should avoid planning an incision that is too small to comfortably accommodate the caliber of the endoscope as ischemia resulting from an inappropriately small incision will place the patient at risk for necrosis and a poor cosmetic result. Injection of local anesthetic into the dermis so as to form a wheal causes a temporary expansion of the skin, which may then be incised with the goal of producing a smaller incision as the wheal resolves and the skin retracts postoperatively. The incision itself should be crafted using a scalpel with minimal use of cautery near the skin as thermal injury to the skin may lead to a suboptimal cosmetic result.

To achieve the best cosmetic result upon closure, a small-diameter resorbable monofilament suture should be employed using a running subcuticular technique. For the typically small incision produced, a buried knot is usually unnecessary and suture ends may be left outside the body using the in-out-in technique at the apices of the incision.

Postoperatively, the wound is kept dry and dressed with a polymer agent such as Dermabond, which reduces skin tension and acts as a semi-occlusive barrier that may be especially helpful in the lumbar spine. This barrier is left undisturbed and can be expected to fall off independently after approximately 2 weeks.

26.5 Mobilization

Early postoperative mobilization is encouraged as it has been shown to improve postoperative pain control and accelerate the return to work.[7] Early mobilization also reduces the risk of pulmonary complications, venous thromboembolism, hospital length of stay, and wound care complications. Generally, for endoscopic spine surgery procedures, no bracing is needed and should be avoided unless necessary to encourage normal mobilization and promote incisional healing.

26.6 Conclusion

The minimally invasive nature of full-endoscopic spine surgery allows for a very well-tolerated postoperative recovery period for patients. However, the surgeon should actively lay the foundations for this postoperative course prior to undertaking any operation. Thoughtfully considering the individual needs of each patient and taking steps to mitigate potential complications related to infection, pain control, functional recovery, and cosmesis will ensure each patient derives the full benefit of full-endoscopic spine surgery.

References

[1] Cizik AM, Lee MJ, Martin BI, et al. Using the spine surgical invasiveness index to identify risk of surgical site infection: a multivariate analysis. J Bone Joint Surg Am. 2012; 94(4):335–342

[2] Shaffer WO, Baisden JL, Fernand R, Matz PG, Society NAS, North American Spine Society. An evidence-based clinical guideline for antibiotic prophylaxis in spine surgery. Spine J. 2013; 13(10):1387–1392

[3] Apfelbaum JL, Chen C, Mehta SS, Gan TJ. Postoperative pain experience: results from a national survey suggest postoperative pain continues to be undermanaged. Anesth Analg. 2003; 97(2):534–540

[4] Lee BH, Park JO, Suk KS, et al. Pre-emptive and multi-modal perioperative pain management may improve quality of life in patients undergoing spinal surgery. Pain Physician. 2013; 16(3):E217–E226

[5] Moonla R, Threetipayarak A, Panpaisarn C, et al. Comparison of preoperative and postoperative parecoxib administration for pain control following major spine surgery. Asian Spine J. 2018; 12(5):893–901

[6] Chang SL. Potential therapeutic strategy to treat substance abuse related disorders. Yao Wu Shi Pin Fen Xi. 2013; 21(4):S25–S26

[7] Daly CD, Lim KZ, Lewis J, et al. Lumbar microdiscectomy and post-operative activity restrictions: a protocol for a single blinded randomised controlled trial. BMC Musculoskelet Disord. 2017; 18(1):312

Appendix: AOSpine Nomenclature System

Type of Procedure	Target area	Principal anatomical landmark
Full-endoscopic diskectomy		
1. Full-endoscopic cervical diskectomy		
• Anterior endoscopic cervical diskectomy (AECD)	Uncinate process	N/A
• Posterior endoscopic cervical diskectomy (PECD)	Juxtaposed edges of index-level laminae	Caudal index-level pedicle
2. Full-endoscopic thoracic diskectomy		
• Transforaminal endoscopic thoracic diskectomy (TETD)	Caudal index level SAP	Caudal index-level pedicle
3. Full-endoscopic lumbar diskectomy		
• Transforaminal endoscopic lumbar diskectomy (TELD)	Medial aspect of the foraminal annular window	Caudal index-level pedicle
• Interlaminar endoscopic lumbar diskectomy (IELD)	Interlaminar window	Yellow ligament
• Extraforaminal endoscopic lumbar diskectomy (EELD)	Superolateral aspect of the caudal index-level pedicle	Foraminal yellow ligament
Full-endoscopic foraminotomy		
• Posterior endoscopic cervical foraminotomy (PECF)	Juxtaposed edges of index-level laminae	Caudal index-level pedicle
• Transforaminal endoscopic lumbar foraminotomy (TELF)	Caudal index level SAP	Caudal index-level pedicle
• Interlaminar endoscopic contralateral lumbar foraminotomy (IECLF)	Spinolaminar junction	Contralateral SAP
Full-endoscopic lumbar lateral recess decompression		
• Transforaminal endoscopic lateral recess decompression (TE-LRD)	Caudal index-level SAP	Caudal index-level pedicle
• Interlaminar endoscopic lateral recess decompression (IE-LRD)	Inferomedial edge of the rostral index-level lamina	Lamina insertion of the yellow ligament
Full-endoscopic laminotomy for bilateral decompression		
• Cervical endoscopic unilateral laminotomy for bilateral decompression (CE-ULBD)	Juxtaposed edges of index-level laminae	Lamina insertion of the yellow ligament
• Thoracic endoscopic unilateral laminotomy for bilateral decompression (TE-ULBD)	Inferomedial edge of the rostral index-level lamina	Lamina insertion of the yellow ligament
• Lumbar endoscopic unilateral laminotomy for bilateral decompression (LE-ULBD)	Inferomedial edge of the rostral index-level lamina	Lamina insertion of the yellow ligament

Abbreviation: SAP, Superior articular process.

Index

Note: Page numbers set **bold** or *italic* indicate headings or figures, respectively.

Index